W9-BZL-597

Natural Posture
for Pain-Free Living

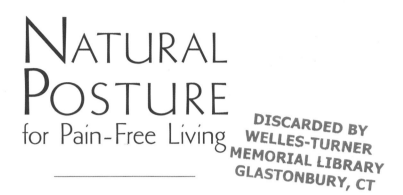

"Never before in the world of fitness has there been a more readable, ground-breaking, or seminal book than *Natural Posture for Pain-Free Living*. Through this revolutionary book, Kathleen Porter is about to rock your world!"

JEAN COUCH, FOUNDER AND DIRECTOR OF THE BALANCE CENTER
AND COAUTHOR OF *THE RUNNER'S YOGA BOOK*

"As a family physician treating my share of patients with back pain, neck pain, osteoporosis, and dysfunctional labor, I find this book instructive. Kathleen Porter's observation of peoples around the world who retain their natural alignment, movement, and relaxation is a clear window into the healing of the chronic pain syndromes of our culture. More than that, her work has been personally transformative."

LEAH MORTON, M.D., FAMILY PRACTITIONER

"In *Natural Posture for Pain-Free Living,* Kathleen Porter powerfully portrays the extensive damage we do to our bodies when we lose connection to natural principles of body alignment. Rather than looking to surgery, medication, and infinite exercise technologies to find freedom from discomfort and pain, we need only learn to stand, sit, walk, and move the way we did as young children when we learned organically to let our bones support us. Porter offers an abundance of useful tools for returning to our natural wisdom and greater body fluidity."

INGRID BACCI, PH.D., AUTHOR OF
THE ART OF EFFORTLESS LIVING AND EFFORTLESS PAIN RELIEF

NATURAL POSTURE
for Pain-Free Living

The Practice of Mindful Alignment

...

KATHLEEN PORTER

Healing Arts Press

Rochester, Vermont • Toronto, Canada

Healing Arts Press
One Park Street
Rochester, Vermont 05767
www.HealingArtsPress.com

Healing Arts Press is a division of Inner Traditions International

Originally published in 2006 by Synergy Books under the title *Ageless Spine, Lasting Health: The Open Secret to Pain-Free Living and Comfortable Aging*

Note to the reader: This book is intended as an informational guide. The remedies, approaches, and techniques described herein are meant to supplement, and not to be a substitute for, professional medical care or treatment. They should not be used to treat a serious ailment without prior consultation with a qualified health care professional.

Library of Congress Cataloging-in-Publication Data
Porter, Kathleen, 1947–
  [Ageless spine, lasting health]
  Natural posture for pain-free living : the practice of mindful alignment / Kathleen Porter.
    p. cm.
  Originally published as: Ageless spine, lasting health. Austin, Tex. : Synergy Books, c2006.
  Summary: "How to restore healthy posture from childhood for relief from chronic pain, easy flexibility, and enduring strength and vitality well into old age"—Provided by publisher.
  Includes bibliographical references and index.
  ISBN 978-1-62055-099-1 (pbk.) — ISBN 978-1-62055-141-7 (e-book)
  1. Posture. 2. Spine—Care and hygiene. 3. Chronic pain—Treatment. I. Title.
  RA781.5.P67 2013
  613.7'8—dc23
                                                                    2012044758

Printed and bound in the United States by Versa Press, Inc.

10 9 8 7 6 5 4 3 2 1

Text design and layout by Virginia Scott Bowman
This book was typeset in Garamond Premier Pro, Gill Sans, Ellington, and Stellar Classic with Arial, Futura, Steller Classic, and Gill Sans used as display typefaces

Grateful acknowledgment is made to the Library of Congress, Wikimedia.org, Shutterstock.com, and iStock.com for use of photographs in this book. Photographs on pages 10 and 12 courtesy of Mary Goodrich; page 37, Alex Feingold (www.math.binghamton.edu/alex); page 122 (top left), Missy and Jeremiah Weismann; page 122 (bottom), Canadian International Learning Foundation (www.canilf.org); page 122 (middle image on right), Andreas Schechner (www.picafric.com); page 185, Halau i ka Wekiu.

To send correspondence to the author of this book, mail a first-class letter to the author c/o Inner Traditions • Bear & Company, One Park Street, Rochester, VT 05767, and we will forward the communication, or contact the author directly at **www.NaturalAlignment.com**.

To Milo, Fiona, Ellery, Tabor, Jay, Talia,
and all children everywhere

■ ■ ■

The miracle is not to walk on water.
The miracle is to walk on the earth in peace.
THICH NHAT HANH

CONTENTS

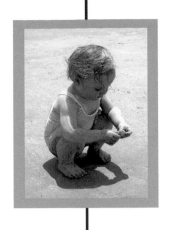

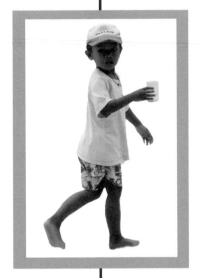

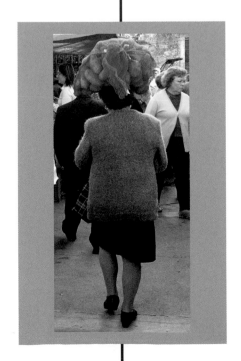

PART ONE
A Body of Knowledge

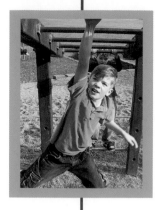

PART TWO
Putting It All Together

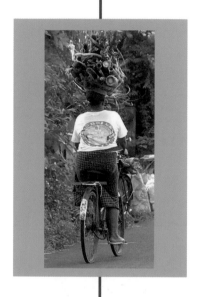

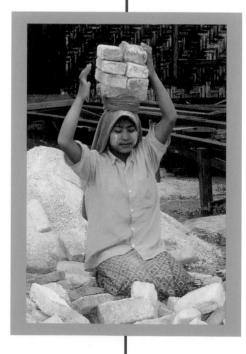

FOREWORD

This is what I know. I know that natural balance is the alignment of the internal skeletal support each human is designed to have. Natural balance yields enormous health benefits to anyone who has the insight to begin. I also know that Kathleen Porter's continuing courage and determination to get this information out to the public is an enormous service.

You may begin this book by looking at the pictures. Just notice the overall shapes of people in balance and out of balance. Ask yourself simple questions—who looks weak, who looks strong? Who is straight, who is curved? When a person is curved what does that do to their natural height. When a person is curved, what might that be doing to the shape of the discs in their spine? Your common sense can guide you to obvious answers that can motivate you to begin. The pictures alone may give you the insight to put you on a new path to health.

All of this, and I haven't even mentioned pain. There are so many benefits of natural balance: moment-to-moment awareness, recovering your natural strength, regaining your natural height, looking like a million dollars, and then there is the relief. The guidelines in this book are enormously powerful, and the first sensations most likely to be perceived are those of relief, feeling better. As you reposition yourself according to the guidelines, you will find that suddenly your muscles can stop holding you up and the tension you are carrying around night and day begins to dissolve. As the bones support you more and more, they are naturally doing the weight lifting that makes them strong. And the great thing is, you don't even have to get this absolutely right, you just have to be in the ballpark.

The book says it all so well. It can give you such a great start; jump in with both feet. Take the plunge.

I would like to again acknowledge with gratitude the brilliance of Noelle Perez, who did all of the original research that has inspired so many of us to take up the torch for each person on the planet to have the option to live in natural balance, and to congratulate Kathleen for clarifying, yet again, why and how to live in natural balance.

JEAN COUCH

■ ■ ■

Jean Couch is the founder and director of the Balance Center, where she has developed methods for teaching concrete guidelines for pain-free posture based on original research by Noelle Perez of Paris, France. More than two decades ago Balance helped Couch eliminate sciatica, back pains, pronounced kyphosis, and a dowager's hump. She has since devoted herself to spreading spinal health and back relief through Balance. The author of *The Runner's Yoga Book,* she teaches workshops and lectures throughout the United States and Canada.

PREFACE

In addition to addressing natural structural alignment, this book also touches on other themes. It is one part anthropology, one part physical therapy, one part textbook, one part travelogue, another part—a very big part, I hope—a plea for research into the health implications related to skeletal alignment.

Many of the photographs were taken by me while traveling in Myanmar (formerly Burma), Thailand, Vietnam, Indonesia, Portugal, and England, as well as in the United States. The rest are photographs taken by others, all selected because they are clear demonstrations of the points being made here. These images show people of varying ages and body types, of multiple ethnic groups and nationalities, and different religious beliefs. The greatest differences among peoples of the world are cultural, geographic, economic, and religious. While far beyond the scope of this book, these differences cannot go unacknowledged. It is easy to romanticize the lives of women who can easily carry heavy loads on their heads while disregarding the often difficult and unfair conditions in which so many people in the world are forced to live and work, conditions frequently caused by such things as the long-term consequences of colonialism and exploitative economic practices.

This point touches on the fact that whenever photographs of unknown people are included in any book or magazine it raises certain ethical questions, no matter how we might try to justify our intentions. While some of the people who were photographed for this book quite willingly gave their permission, others did not have an opportunity to make that choice. I hope it is true that many people will be helped by reading this book and viewing these images—indeed that is my motivation for writing this—but I am not thoroughly satisfied with this ends-justifies-the-means reasoning. I wish to extend my gratitude to all the people whose images I have gathered here. I encourage anyone reading this to recognize the humanity of the people inside these photographs rather than only seeing them as examples.

I take full responsibility for the choices I have made here and sincerely hope that I have caused no harm.

American culture is difficult to define; we are such a diverse and multi-ethnic collection of people. Some Americans, because of their heritage or certain childhood influences, are less likely to be susceptible to conditioned beliefs and characteristics of the dominant culture, such as tucking the butt or sucking in the belly. By *dominant culture* I mean the one that is almost single-mindedly promoted by mainstream media through television, magazines, and movies, as well as a steady bombardment of other messages we absorb in countless ways every day. This dominant culture sets the standard and spells out what is attractive, healthy, fit, and acceptable while establishing deeply embedded beliefs in the psyches of many people in America today. Generally these rules, though unconsciously mandated, are a departure from what is natural and healthy. An example of this is the commonly subscribed-to belief that says that women, in order to be attractive, must have flat bellies.

The words *we, our,* and *us* are sometimes used in this book to refer to those who tend to be unconsciously conditioned and influenced by these mainstream messages. I put myself and almost everyone else in this country in that category. In other cases, *we* is used to refer to everyone's membership in the global human melting pot. Hoping that I have succeeded in making these distinctions clear within these pages, I leave it to the reader to determine how the use of *we* is intended in the context of any given passage.

One last note: A commonly held belief is the notion that less labor and greater wealth lead to a better life. Some people see physical labor as demeaning, as being delegated to a lower place on the status scale. After all, you don't need an advanced degree to dig a trench or build a rock wall. What is often overlooked is that some people take great joy in physical labor, especially those whose bodies move naturally, with ease of movement and the enjoyment of innate strength and flexibility. At the end of a day's work they may feel less worn out than someone who struggled to sit comfortably at a desk all day and then fought traffic to get home. Indeed, upward mobility can often spell the end of natural mobility. Even people who regularly exercise and work out in the hopes of counteracting a sedentary lifestyle will often pay someone else to mow their lawns.

I sometimes imagine what it would be like to live in a society where citizens engage physically in community life by helping their elderly neighbors clean leaves from their gutters, by actively playing with their children at the playground, by growing food in large, thriving community gardens, and by participating as part-ners alongside local government workers to maintain the roadsides and public facilities. The life of the body can be integrated so easily into the life of a vibrant community, combining physical exercise (done in alignment!) with activities that breathe enlivenment into our society, preserve and enhance our environment, and build connections with our own selves and each other.

ACKNOWLEDGMENTS

After traveling the solitary and sometimes lonely road of self-publishing this book, it was pure joy to have the assistance and dedication of an entire talented team working together to bring this new revised edition to life. My agent, Deanna Leah, started this wonderful ball rolling, and Jon Graham at Inner Traditions, along with Jeanie Levitan, Jamaica Burns Griffin, Elizabeth Wilson, Manzanita Carpenter, Peri Ann Swan, Virginia Scott Bowman, and support staff shepherded it across the finish line. Throughout this process, I have been in their highly capable hands, for which I, and the reader, can be grateful!

Evan Ing worked alongside me for hours on end, offering his multiple talents in upgrading and organizing the photographs and illustrations. He managed to save the day, yet again.

For a healthy number of decades now, I have been the beneficiary of the wisdom and guidance of many brilliant teachers who have held my hand, pointed the way, and even given a not-so-gentle kick down this road. I especially want to single out Jean Couch, who has given generously and worked single-mindedly all these years to empower people with the resources for knowing how to heal their own pain. Noelle Perez laid a foundation so large and solid that Jean and many others, myself included, have been able to add an ever-evolving structure that is destined to change our understanding of how the body is designed to work.

I am blessed by friendships, family ties and professional associations that, woven together, sustain me with continuous acceptance, encouragement, and support. I thank my lucky stars that I have been brought together in this life with Thea Beckett, Irene McNeely, Patra Conley, Kathryn Grout, Patricia Salmon, Wendell Ing, Kenneth Lahti, Jan Cooper, Carter Beckett, Jacob Trubin, Elaine Lee, Cindy Berry, Sally Mermel, Jeffrey Mermel, Anne Marie Claire, Rhona Klein, Jill Schatten, Rebecca Erickson, Betty Lee, Tabor Bergh, Stacey Tripeny, Sally Ho, Ira Ono, Sandra Pickard, Anne Kokubun, Russell Kokubun, Linda Haynes,

Wendy Thomas-Miyamoto, Moline Whitson, Norman Skinner, Kristin Porter, Jack Nguyen, Diane McChesney Parfitt, Nancy Morgan, Barb Isham, Cindy Debus, Patti Chikasuye, Colleen Ziroli, Diane Li, Marianne Kuipers Tilanus, Hettie Schofield, Ho Sheng Chi, Milo Jarvis, Karen Umehara, Sherry Genauer, Gabe Genauer, Lorna Larson-Jeyte, Cynee Wenner, Marilyn Nicholson, Kathleen Golden, Peter Golden, Dianne Horwitz, Dawn Pung, Tanya Paltin, Sam Paltin, Maria Jaramillo, Barbara Heintz, Billy Sammons, Joanne Hunter, Carol Cohan, Mary Copenhaver, Daralynn Higgins, Sharon Kaneshiro Mols, Kaila Kukla, Susan Buswell, Avigail Roberg, Arline Krieger, and elementary school teachers extraordinaire, Kaholo Daguman, Kathy Wines, and Jeff Rood.

My beautiful family continues to grace my life with their love, patience, and unending goodwill. I love you Meredith Ing, Kendra Ing, Evan Ing, Wendell Ing, Evan Bissell, Weston Willard, Israel Sims, and Milo Heuluokaha`i Willard.

INTRODUCTION

THE STATE OF HUMAN health today is in full-blown crisis. Not only is the American health care system broken, but our bodies are also broken. The causes are many, but I believe the primary reason for this is the wholesale disconnection occurring between humans and the natural world. We have forgotten that each and every one of us is as much a part of nature as the bird that flies across the sky and the cheetah that pursues a meal at lightning speed. Humans are given the same potential as any species to come into the world with all the physical resources we need to live our lives empowered by a design that, under normal circumstances, works and moves with ease for a whole lifetime, free from strain or pain. As with all other creatures, the human design is specific to our particular needs and requirements, one of which is our unique ability to walk upright. Until recently this had been a bonus more than it was a problem, but modernization and technological advancement of our culture, and the accompanying habits of being more sedentary and sitting poorly, have set new patterns in place, sometimes from a very young age, that are causing problems for millions of people.

Intact indigenous cultures are likely to feel this connection to the earth through bodies that align along the axis and are thus open to an energetic exchange between the body and the earth. The scientific explanation for this is ground reaction force (GRF) as it relates to Newton's third law of motion: for every action, there is an equal and opposite reaction. Healthy newborn babies, when lying on their stomachs, discover this when pushing down onto the surface on which they are lying. If they did not, they would never be able to raise their heads. At first the push is small, and the equal reaction beneath their skin is small too. Gradually, as this process builds the strength that allows them to push harder, a deep core response grows within the body that is equal to that stronger push. Engaging with the earth in this way guides the infant, over a number of months, from a state of helplessness and powerlessness to soon being a fully enlivened toddler able to run and jump for the joy of being a body. For many children today this connection is broken in the earliest months of life. This is a tragedy. The chapter in this book that addresses what is happening with children today has been revised and updated to include expanded information about this. I am convinced that, as we finally begin to understand these concepts, it will come to light that some, if not most, of the neurodevelopmental problems plaguing children in epidemic numbers today come from the disruption of what, in normal development, is a natural unfolding of an essential and primal process.

Eight years ago, when I first wrote this book, I struggled to find an agent or a publisher who would take this on. Posture, I was told, was not a subject that would sell. Try as I might to explain this was oh so much more than a book *just* about posture, no one was buying it. It seemed that as long as people could take a yoga class, work out at the gym, lie on a massage table, or pay a visit to the chiropractor, this was all that was needed to manage the tension and pain that most of us had come to believe are simply inconvenient features that come with having a body.

Being a body, however, turns out to be something very different from just having one. *Natural Posture for Pain-Free Living* is a book about integrating what it means to *have a body* that is governed by the physical rules that apply to everything in our world with how to *be a body* that is anchored in mindfulness and a quality of felt presence. The joining of these two aspects of being physically human is more likely to provide us with the satisfying experience of being pain-free, easily flexible, genuinely strong, full of vitality, and deeply aware—perhaps best described as embodied presence.

Much has changed since I self-published the first edition of this book. Interest in this subject has grown tremendously, partly as a result of the fact that in spite of (and sometimes because of) all the hours spent stretching and strengthening muscles, many people are *still* in pain. It has taken a long time for many of us to begin to recognize that if the knee hurts, it might have something to do with how the bones in the feet are positioned; and if the neck hurts, maybe the problem lies with whether the pelvis is able to support an aligned spine on top of which the head can balance freely, without having to be held in place by tense muscles. In our muscle-obsessed society we have forgotten that the musculoskeletal system is a partnership of muscles and bones. By not recognizing the skeleton's key role in providing underlying, aligned support, we force our muscles to make up for this deficit by imposing dysfunctional patterns of use on them in everything they do.

I have been privileged to have worked with many people who have shown me how readily chronic pain can be relieved by *relearning* how to align their bones and engage the deepest core of internal support. The emphasis is on relearning, because this alignment is what almost all of us first discovered as well-developing babies and toddlers. Many people have experienced total recovery from long-standing problems after a long list of other approaches failed to bring lasting relief. This was true even in instances where people had been told they needed surgery to correct a problem in their backs, necks, knees, or hips. Some people *do* need surgery and receive great benefit from it, so it's important to be clear here that what we are talking about is not a cure-all. Even so, I believe, barring accidents, most orthopedic surgeries could be avoided if the body's natural alignment is never lost in the first place.

I once would have thought this to be a simplistic, overblown claim before I came upon a body education and movement technique called Balance. When I first met Jean Couch, the founder of the Balance Center, I was a massage therapist and yoga teacher with a rigorous practice who was continually plagued with recurring tension in my neck and shoulders and a back condition that could be relieved only by daily stretching. Unfortunately, stretching sometimes aggravated a hip that was unstable and popped out of alignment in certain positions and activities, which was followed by days (and sleepless nights) of nagging pain.

In spite of the fact that for a number of years I had taught other people how to relax, proving the adage that you teach what you need to know, I held on to varying amounts of tension in my body and my mind. I was generally unaware at the time that I was doing this. I also didn't realize that I had become addicted to stretching and working out. After all, wasn't I doing what other conscious people were doing—taking care of myself by working at staying fit? Stretching and sweating away tension felt so good and gave me such relief that I never questioned why the tension returned again so quickly or why I had to repeat my exercise regimen on a daily basis in order to feel good enough. Whenever I skipped the stretching for any reason, the aches and pains returned in no time at all.

Today a growing number of people in the United States and Europe have been working to develop a new field of study, or body of knowledge, that has grown out of the pioneering work of Noelle Perez. First inspired by the teachings of her mentor, B. K. S. Iyengar, with whom she began studying in 1959, Perez researched principles of the body's natural alignment along the vertical axis of gravity through the observation of indigenous people around the world. Perez went on to establish l'Institute Superior d'Aplomb in Paris, France. Other pioneers of body mechanics, including F. M. Alexander, Mabel Ellsworth Todd, Charlotte Selver, and Ida Rolf, contributed invaluable insights into how the natural body is designed for comfort and ease of movement. Additionally, long-established approaches to movement and martial arts such as qigong, t'ai chi, aikido, and indigenous and traditional dance forms, when practiced in their original form, have served to reinforce the natural mechanical movements of the body. The principles of natural alignment described here are not at odds with these practices, or vice versa. All of these practices, when done correctly, are beneficial to almost anyone. The basis for the information presented here, however, is founded on details pertaining to natural balance as originally described by Noelle Perez. My own particular emphasis relative to this information is on the essential role of an aligned skeleton as the underlying framework of support for everything; the functioning of muscles that are attached to those bones and the efficiency of all the working parts of all the body's systems. I believe this alignment explains why approaches to movement and body awareness such as qigong, t'ai chi, yoga, and the Alexander technique can be so effective in relieving pain and promoting ease of movement. When done correctly, these approaches reinforce the body's natural design and promote its homeostatic center.

While it is unlikely any of these methods will ever be taught in medical schools, it is my hope that one day the body's natural skeletal alignment will be recognized as the structural basis for all-around good health and will be a key part of the curriculum for medical students, physical therapists, and other health practitioners. Right now the actual relationship of skeletal bones to each other is overlooked and misunderstood, but when this catches on at long last, many dramatic and positive changes will occur.

Principles of natural alignment do not, in themselves, represent a specific technique or method, although some of us who are working with this information, myself included, are developing our own unique approaches to sharing these concepts (for further details, see the resources section at the end of the book). Jean Couch calls what she teaches Balance, Dana Davis calls it Body Balance, Angie Thusius calls it Kentro, Esther Gokhale calls it the Gokhale method, and Lisa Ann McCall has developed the McCall method. I have developed a program I call Mindful Alignment that emphasizes the role of mindfulness in putting these principles into practice. More simply, what we are all talking about is *natural alignment*. There are others too, each one of them spawned by the original work of Noelle Perez. The bottom line is that this must be based, thoroughly and completely, on the natural biomechanical design inherent to the human species. Anything other than an approach that describes and promotes these very specific details of alignment does not meet the criteria for natural alignment.

Ideas for how to impart this information are continuously evolving as we experience profound changes in ourselves as well as witnessing them in others who practice this. Often, when I observe people, I imagine them attached to puppet strings or envision interior wheels turning. I've created images of these things, not only as a way to help people understand and learn this information but also as a way to help promote these ideas and inspire research.

While the details of the instructions for learning this may vary among the different methods, each approach must be, at the bottom line, solidly based on the natural human alignment that is discovered by naturally developing toddlers everywhere—namely, alignment that is innate to the human species. In fact, by inhabiting the body this way we acknowledge that we are fully and genuinely creatures of nature, just like all other creatures that inhabit this Earth.

Remarkably, there is no research that I am aware of that examines aspects of health in adults or children that is based on these very specific details of natural skeletal alignment. This represents a serious oversight in a world where the prescription pad is often the first line of defense in addressing a long list of health issues of unknown cause.

The more we understand our own body's anatomy as it relates to basic mechanics and natural movement, the better we can know how to guide our own process of healing from the inside out. Thus I have included many details—too many for some readers—about how the body works and moves. My goal is to empower the student with the tools needed to become one's own best teacher. After all, when it comes to inhabiting a body with awareness, it is, unquestionably, an inside job. At the center of our physical being is an energetic core that anchors us to the Earth and provides the stability for us to be upright. Skeletal alignment is the framework on which this stability is constructed. It is what healthy babies discover all on their own and what they will carry with them throughout their lives, provided it is not disrupted and lost.

In writing and talking about this, I've sometimes questioned using words such as the *intention of the human design*. As hard as I've tried, I have not been able to find other words that match what I am trying to say. Please note that when these words are used here they strictly mean a design that conforms to and grows out from mechanical, scientific, and natural laws of physics as they pertain to matter, motion, energy, force, mathematics, and gravity. These design rules explain the *how* of a small person who is able to carry an enormously heavy load of rocks on the head with ease, or the *why* of cartilage in a knee joint that wears out when the knee is repeatedly bent while medially rotated. One underlying philosophy at odds with this human design, however, is the notion that we are somehow apart *from,* rather than a part *of,* this natural world. This belief has resulted in an environmental crisis of breathtaking magnitude that simultaneously drives the separation from our own natural state of good health.

Such denial of the Earth as home sometimes comes out of a belief that we are simply an enduring soul or spirit and nothing more. "You are not your body" and "we must transcend the body" are oft-repeated themes in various spiritual practices. While these concepts may have meaning in an ultimate philosophical sense, they can present serious problems for anyone living everyday life as a human being, right here, right now. Try having a spiritual experience, no matter how elevated and lofty, without a body. There may be moments in time when we experience being transported beyond the body to a realm of existence that might be described by some as union with God or pure consciousness. As long as we are living, breathing human beings, this body exists as the physical seat of such experiences. When such transcendent states of mind occur, at least for most of us, they are fleeting. What is not fleeting, however, is the deeply felt sense of connection between our bodies and this Earth that is available every waking moment when our bodies abide by governing physical laws. When we do not conform to these laws, a sense of disconnection as well as chronic tension, pain, and poor health are often the result.

Remarkably, the most common cause of tension and pain in the body—postural misalignment—is thoroughly misunderstood by almost everyone in technologically advanced places in the world. It turns out that our widely accepted belief about what constitutes good posture is based on faulty information that leads to much of the pain we experience. This mistaken view is so widespread in our society and so thoroughly entrenched in our bodies and our minds that it pervades almost every system of exercise, almost every belief about fitness, and many of the messages we receive from doctors and other health professionals, exercise teachers, and sports coaches.

No one is at fault for this. Such is the way of cultural conditioning, where a collective hypnosis takes hold over the course of many years and puts nearly everyone under a spell based on mistaken assumptions. In our current cultural milieu many of our beliefs about health and fitness are built on what we have been taught. Parents, teachers, role models, TV shows, movies, advertising, magazine covers—all of these have been shaped by the same misunderstanding of how our human bodies are designed to work. This belief says that muscular strength, or tension, is what holds us up straight. The unfortunate outcome of this misperception separates many of us from knowing the reality of our biomechanical design. An inner knowing that is our inheritance as humans, as well as an important key to good health and comfortable aging, remains hidden from most of us.

Our relationship with our bodies is ruled by myths that take us ever further from our body's natural design. Prominent among these myths is the as-yet-unchallenged belief that strong *rectus abdominis* muscles, or six-pack abs, are not only necessary to support our backs, but they must be firm in order for us to be attractive, by a culturally dictated standard. This standard says we must conform to an ideal appearance that may have little to do with what is natural or healthy for any particular individual. Millions of people in our society are dedicating themselves to a quest for a body that is sculpted in ways that can be customized in order to have the "body you've always wanted." This gives us the message that our own normal healthy body, within a range of a certain number of pounds, when inhabited with alignment and ease of movement, is not already perfect. In American culture today, where the perceived reflection in the mirror defines our value, most of us find ourselves in the same boat, unaware that the boat is sinking.

This fact became quite obvious to me when I traveled to countries where the conditioned habits are vastly different and where far fewer people have given in to the suck-and-tuck anomaly. These naturally aligned people are mostly found in rural locations or among older populations, with bodies that still function much the same way they did when they were young children first learning how to sit, stand, and bend. Children instinctively know how to be natural, and all healthy children, no matter where in the world they are born, teach themselves how to sit up, stand, and move by organizing themselves (and their bones) around the central axis that aligns with their body's natural center of gravity. Naturally developing babies and toddlers are the gurus for how to live in relaxed, aligned bodies.

The importance of natural structural support cannot be overstated. Structural support is no less important to a human body than properly placed posts, joists, and struts are to a building, no less important than the precise functioning of timing belts, valves, and pistons are to a car engine—indeed, no less important than a trunk is to a tree. The integrity of our structure is not only crucial to our being comfortable and pain-free, it also contributes to many aspects of our overall health and well-being. The natural placement of our bones in any activity and movement determines whether vital energy—the very pulse of life itself—flows freely through our bodies or is blocked and stagnant. The former leads to vibrant health; the latter, to pain and disorder.

Too often naturalness is viewed as an outdated, antiquated concept. The argument that we can't go back to the cave misses the point that in spite of today's high-tech, high-performance world, we are still creatures of nature who are absolutely and wholly dependent on this Earth. We deny this connection at our peril. Living in natural bodies has nothing to do with turning back the clock and everything to do with living in this present moment, with an acceptance of who we really are, right now. An awareness of our physical nature and what it means is an important key to good health, to a sense of well-being, and, ultimately, to finding peace inside our own skin.

Incorporated into this new edition are exercises that allow you to "Try It On!" while you are reading the information being presented. Also included in this new edition is a chapter on how to practice yoga safely. Yoga provides many wonderful benefits when it is practiced in accordance with the body's natural design. Unfortunately it can, and often does, create problems for bodies with deeply embedded patterns of misalignment. A new chapter called "Yoga on the Axis" has been added that includes simple instructions that anchor the body and stabilize the core. Written in collaboration with Moline Whitson, who is successfully incorporating these principles into her classes at Harmony Yoga in Portland, Oregon, this chapter offers guidelines to ensure that practicing yoga is safe, regardless of whatever limitations one might have. Once learned, these instructions can be applied in other *asana,* or yoga positions, as well.

It will be a new day when principles of natural alignment have found wide acceptance as the basis for how the human body works. Alignment not only refers to the skeleton organizing itself around the vertical axis of gravity but also to each one of us aligning ourselves with a basic truth of our physical nature.

Before this can happen, research must show—and it is only a matter of time before it will—that alignment along the vertical axis and the solid core of support this generates are necessary ingredients for being optimally healthy. As such, this information will finally be an accepted part of everyday health care, providing doctors and other health professionals with tools for empowering their patients to heal themselves whenever possible.

The best outcome of all will be when healthier people, as a matter of course, directly experience their connection with the Earth through a body that conforms to its physical laws. They will know themselves to be part of a whole made up of many parts, of which they—*we*—are one. Knowing this, we will quite naturally care for this Earth and all its species in the same way we will care for ourselves and each other.

PART ONE

■ ■ ■

A Body of Knowledge

My body
you are so kind
to sit and wait for me
while I am away

I wander off
but you don't budge
When I return
to my true home
it is you

CASEY HAYDEN

DESIGN FOR LIFE

WHO IS MORE FIT? Is it a small woman with elastic muscles and naturally aligned bones or a much larger man with six-pack abs and firmly developed pecs, deltoids, and biceps?

The small woman pictured here is able to carry heavy rocks on her head all day long, day after day, without strain. Because the weight of the load is distributed

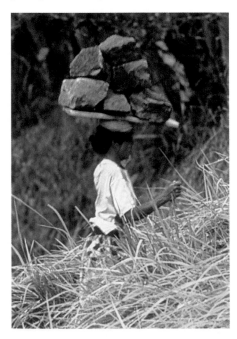

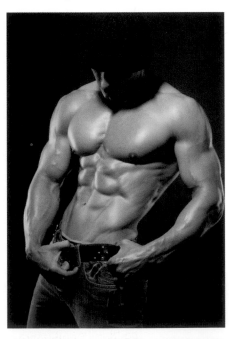

Despite her small size, this woman exhibits incredible strength thanks to her naturally aligned bones and elastic muscles.

This man's strength lies in his muscles alone rather than in the integration of fully functioning parts. Muscles that have been developed this way are storehouses of contracted tension.

through aligned bones, the bones actually do the work of carrying the load. Her muscles are thus free to perform their primary job of moving the bones without strain. In this scenario the musculoskeletal system functions as a dynamic interplay between bones and muscles that requires that the bones be aligned and the muscles be elastic. This balanced interplay is the hallmark of true fitness.

This man is clearly strong in ways the woman is not. His power lies within his muscles alone, not in an overall integrated whole of fully functioning parts. The popular culture of fitness today is partly based on the idea that developed muscles are a requirement of fitness. Unfortunately muscles that have been developed in this way are storehouses of contracted tension, making it difficult for them to lengthen and relax. This type of strength must be worked at continuously and is dependent on a regular maintenance routine. This man's spine is shortened and compressed. His breathing is restricted because of a diaphragm that doesn't move in a natural, efficient way. The range of motion of his shoulders and hips is greatly restricted. It is ironic that the strength he has worked so hard to acquire has also become a type of weakness.

Unnatural strength
- has its power in purposely developed muscles,
- must be continuously worked at to be maintained,
- limits the range of motion of the joints,
- restricts elasticity of the diaphragm, and
- compresses the spine.

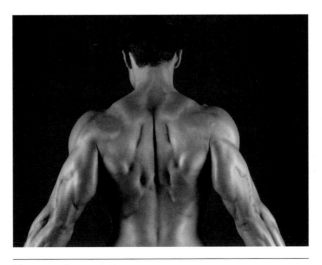

Unnatural strength

Natural strength

- has its power in aligned bones,
- is innate and reinforced in ordinary activities,
- promotes natural, easy flexibility of joints, and
- elongates the spine.

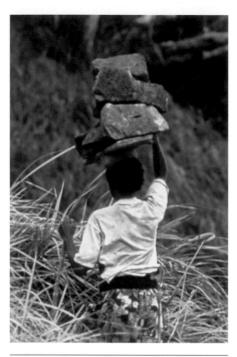

Natural strength

THE NORMALIZATION OF PAIN

The modern-day confusion about what constitutes authentic strength and natural, easy flexibility is at the root of most of the chronic pain experienced by millions of people every day. In the United States today millions of people live with chronic aches and pains that severely limit their activities, affect their ability to work, cost them thousands of dollars in lost wages, and impair their enjoyment of life. Employers, insurance companies, and workers' compensation funds pay billions of dollars each year for lost time on the job and benefits to injured employees.

Whether pain is chronic and low level or severe and debilitating, it has become an enormous problem in our country. In fact, pain is so commonplace it has come to be considered a normal fact of life. The epidemic of chronic pain has given way to a new medical specialty—pain management—because it is assumed that, in many cases, pain is something one simply must learn to live with. Too often pain management relies on the use of prescription drugs that generate many billions of dollars in profits for pharmaceutical companies while driving a crippling addiction problem for millions of Americans.

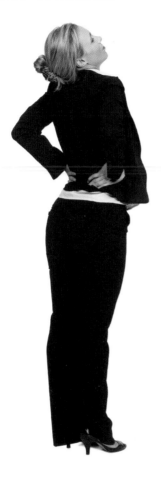

Pain, whether chronic and low level or severe and debilitating, has become an enormous problem in our country.

The list of complaints is long and includes general unexplained lower back pain, hip and knee pain, arthritis, tendonitis, sciatica, fibromyalgia, plantar fasciitis, frozen shoulder, rotator cuff injury, herniated or bulging discs, degenerative disc disease, spinal stenosis, spondylolisthesis, temporomandibular joint disorder (TMJ), and chronic tension in neck and shoulder muscles. Much of this pain appears to be idiopathic, meaning it has no clear, discernible cause, making it difficult for doctors to know how to treat it. When asked what caused their pain, people will often say things such as, "I shouldn't have lifted that box of books," or "I've been running for twenty years, and my knees finally wore out," or "I'm not as young as I used to be."

If any of these people knew what their bodies were actually telling them they might respond with more accurate answers. They might say, "Bending to lift a box of books, my pelvis was tucked under, causing my back to round and preventing my core from stabilizing my spine. This forced my back to strain rather than being able to rely on aligned bones working with the strength of my legs and arms to do the work." Or one might say, "Running for twenty years with misaligned bones has put persistent stress on my knees, causing the cartilage to wear out." Or possibly the response might be, "This aging body is now paying the price for not living according to its natural design."

It can be startling to discover that exercise, in and of itself and in spite of its obvious benefits, is seldom the solution for this kind of pain over the long run. In fact, because exercise can reinforce and embed unhelpful patterns of movement, it can, and often does, cause the pain in the first place. Eventually we all pay the price if our bones have not been able to do the job of supporting us throughout the years.

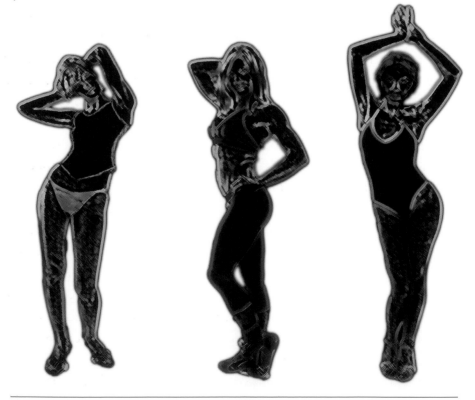

By reinforcing and embedding unhelpful patterns of movement, exercise can, and often does, cause people's pain. For many people today, fitness has become more about how one looks than how one feels.

Musculoskeletal pain is far less of a problem in some parts of the world, even in places where people do a lot of manual labor for years on end.[1] The secret seems to be that some people never lose the biomechanical principles of the human design, something all healthy toddlers discover when first learning how to stand and walk.

The dictionary definition of the popularized word *fitness* describes it to mean "possessing a quality of strength and overall health." Nevertheless, for many people today fitness has become more about how one looks than how one feels. This is a cultural standard that has nothing to do with what is natural to our species' design.

In our popular quest for fitness and a culturally imposed standard of beauty, many of us unwittingly disregard the importance of skeletal alignment and create conditions that compromise our long-term health. A misaligned skeleton causes muscles that attach to the skeleton to either shorten or lengthen unnaturally. This creates chronic tension that restricts mobility of certain joints. It also impairs breathing, compresses vertebrae, puts pressure on and distorts the spinal cord (the primary neural pathway), and affects circulation. It would be hard to argue with the fact that all of these factors have far-reaching consequences for one's health.

Fitness becomes something other than what we thought it was when we apply it to an older woman who is clearly "out of shape" by our cultural standards yet easily carries fifty pounds of potatoes on her head (see photo on the following page). Many people who regularly work out at the gym would feel a strain in their backs or necks if they tried to do this. It is probably a safe bet that the woman carrying the potatoes on her head does not practice yoga or Pilates, jog, or participate in any other type of formal exercise. Her strength is of a different sort than simply the muscular kind that has to be acquired through time and effort. Her strength is bone deep and comes from a skeleton that has never changed its alignment from the time she was a young child. Her strength is neither superficial (concentrated in muscles close to the surface of her body) nor is it artificial.

In America today upward of 80 percent of people suffer back pain and seek treatment at some point, be it chiropractic, massage, physical therapy, Rolfing, acupuncture, epidural injections, pain medication, or surgery. The total cost of treating people who suffer back pain tops $100 billion a year.[2] The incidence of

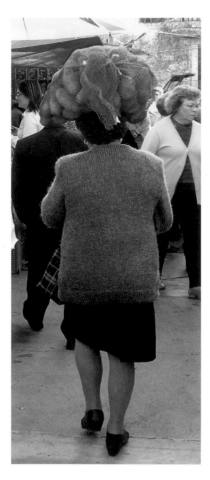

By our cultural standards this woman may be "out of shape," yet see how easily she carries fifty pounds of potatoes on her head.

back pain drops dramatically in those places where people do not sit at desks all day or regularly use cars and computers or watch television. It is important to note, however, that it is not one's level of activity that determines whether one will experience back pain but, rather, the position of the bones in relationship to each other. Someone who sits with ease for long periods of time with the support of aligned bones may be far better off than someone who is physically active much of the time, if (and this is a very important *if*) the more active person is moving with chronic misalignment of the skeleton. This is because the alignment of the skeleton dictates whether muscles will work in a way that is natural, efficient, and, ultimately, pain-free or in a way that is prone to injury and pain.

Most people who experience chronic pain would just like to feel more comfortable. It can be hard to imagine there could be a correlation between one person carrying a heavy load on her head and someone else getting rid of chronic back pain. Yet each requires the same particular skeletal alignment that conforms to

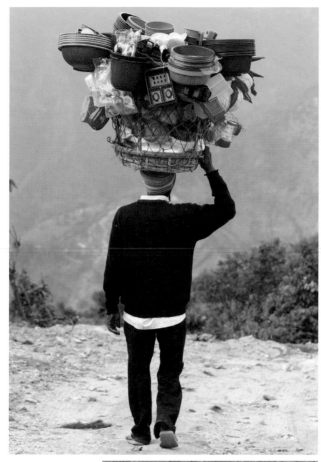

It is not one's level of activity that determines whether one will experience back pain but, rather, the position of the bones in relationship to each other.

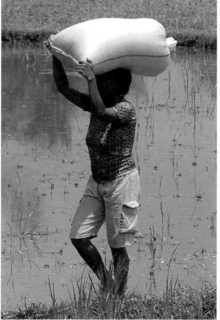

The alignment of the skeleton dictates whether muscles will work in a way that is natural, efficient, and, ultimately, pain-free or in a way that is prone to injury and pain.

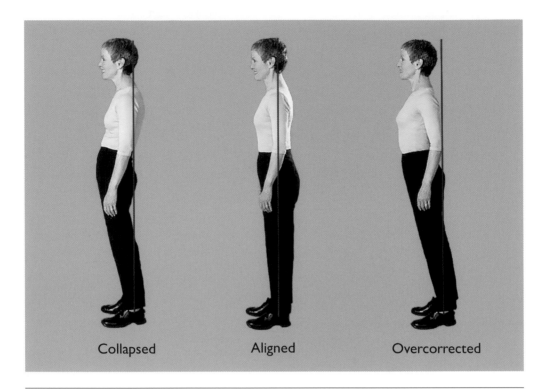

Collapsed   Aligned   Overcorrected

It's easy to see how the collapsed body on the left and the overcorrected body on the right are pulled out of alignment, while the body in the middle is almost perfectly divided in half by the centerline.

natural laws. You certainly don't have to carry a heavy load on your head to heal back pain (in fact, it is advised that you *not* do so), yet the same alignment of bones required to do this successfully is the secret to many people healing chronic pain. Even lifting weights and otherwise working out cannot prepare someone to carry a heavy load on the head if the arrangement of bones in relationship to each other does not conform to natural laws. Indeed, muscle development can interfere with a quality of relaxed strength that is essential for living in a comfortable, pain-free body.

The red lines on the three figures above all start at the ankle and rise up along the vertical axis. It's easy to see how two of these bodies are pulled off the line, while the body in the middle is almost perfectly divided in half by the centerline. The bones in this body are symmetrically arranged around the axis, providing the same solid structural stability required of buildings and all mechanical constructions. Most people in technologically developed places move toward one end of the spectrum or the other, to varying degrees, although rarely do we inhabit the solid, comfortable middle, where the legs serve as vertical columns of support, and the spine is perfectly aligned and optimally elongated.

> The question now begging to be answered by comprehensive research is this: Can someone be truly fit if the bones of the skeleton do not support the body, causing the muscles to be distorted and struggle to compensate, and the spine (the nervous system) is not aligned along the central axis?

HOW CULTURE AFFECTS THE PHYSICAL

Inherited body type and other genetic traits, personal habits, injuries, physical and emotional trauma, patterns of movement, and types and levels of activity are all factors that determine the shape we have as well as the shape we are in. At a very young age we begin to unconsciously become imprinted by the postures, gestures, styles, and tensions of those around us. Before long we become adolescents and may start to acquire the gestures of our friends and idols. Perhaps, without realizing it, we take on a defiant stance by pumping ourselves up like a rooster, or we attempt to withdraw, literally, by collapsing into ourselves in an attempt to become invisible. For many people these early habits set the tone for a whole lifetime, thus affecting our relationship with ourselves and with others, and affecting our long-term health.

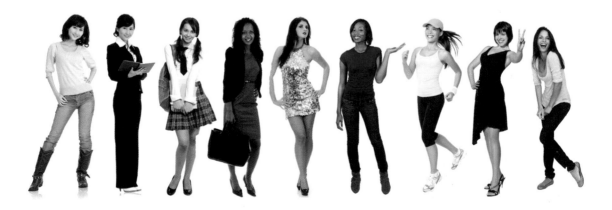

At a very young age we begin to unconsciously become imprinted by the postures, gestures, styles, and tensions of those around us.

Most of us are unaware of the extent to which our self-image and the posture we adopt is defined for us by others. This has been especially true for women. Aside from the cultural expectations put on women that they should strive, above all, to (a) be thin and (b) look young, women seem to have a number of acceptable options for how to inhabit their bodies. Unlike men, it's okay for a woman to appear shy and self-deprecating or coy and seductive. She can also be boldly sexual, wholesomely athletic, assertively confident, or just plain natural. All are familiar ways a woman in our culture might present herself to the world at various times. Each one of the women pictured above has a particular arrangement of skeletal bones that give shape, literally, to the physical persona she is modeling.

Photographs of early North American life, beginning with the earliest Native Americans and including peoples from other countries who came to live in the United States, reveal many naturally aligned bodies. Historical photographs show that many people, up until the early part of the twentieth century, lived with their skeletons lined up along the natural plumb line. While the style of dress was far more formal back then, sometimes giving an impression of rigidity or stiffness, the people pictured on the facing page, while noticeably upright, have the support of aligned bones that allows them to be, in actuality, quite relaxed.

Many cultural changes have occurred during the past century, with remarkable advances in many areas, that include a refreshingly less formal way of dress and an acceptance of differing lifestyle options. Unfortunately, more casual ways of living include widespread physical collapse. A glimpse inside a photo album today reveals bodies that are rarely supported by aligned bones (see page 22). We tend to think this is what relaxing looks like, but this kind of distortion puts considerable stress on the body, forcing some muscles to work hard just to compensate for this lack of underlying support. For the most part, even when people are trying to sit or stand up straight, their pelvis is seldom an anteriorly rotated anchor, making it unable to support the spine.

Changing fashions and shifting fads have played a part in some of the new ways of inhabiting the body over the past one hundred years. Now, in the twenty-first century, so many people are suffering cultural memory loss that we have completely forgotten what the natural carriage of a healthy woman looks like and how inherently capable she is of standing on her own two feet (in this case, vertical legs). A truly healthy woman does not have to work at becoming strong; she simply *is* that way. The more she aligns herself, literally and figuratively, with who she is as a natural human being, the more she brings forward her inherent qualities of

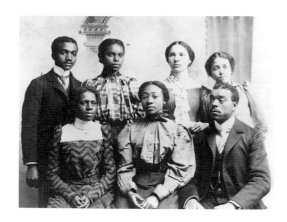
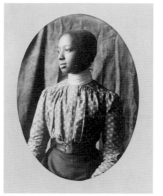
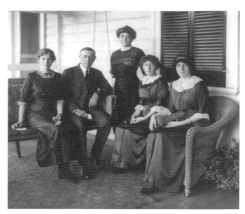

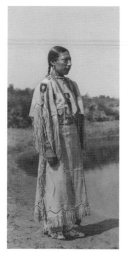
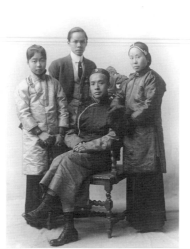
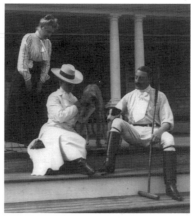
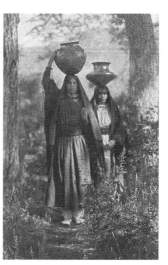

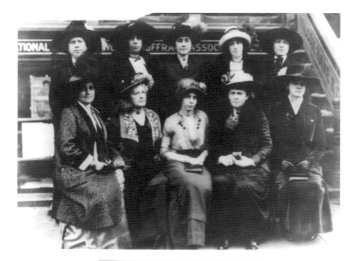
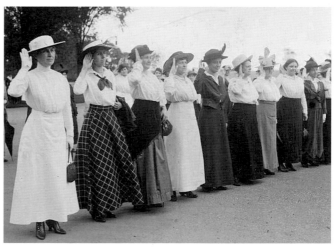

Historical photographs show that while the style of dress was more formal and rigid a hundred years ago, the people had the support of aligned bones, allowing them to be quite relaxed.

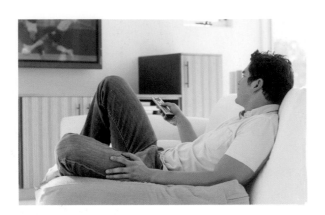

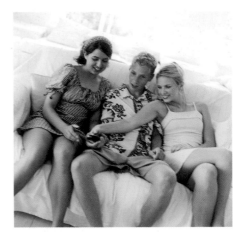

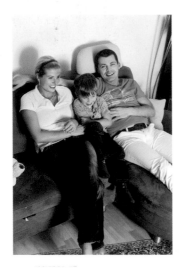

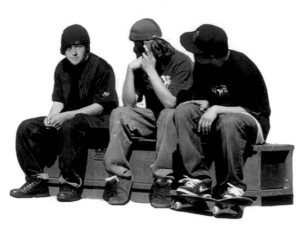

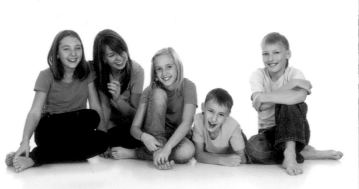

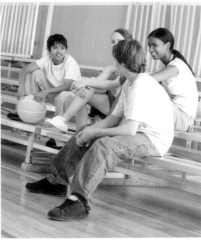

Unfortunately, more casual ways of living have included widespread physical collapse. Notice how the bodies in these pictures lack the support of aligned bones.

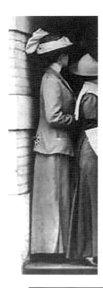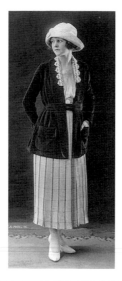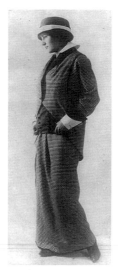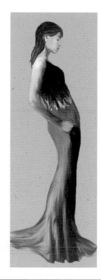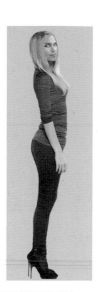

Changing fashions and shifting fads over the past hundred years have played a part in new ways of inhabiting the body.

authentic strength, easy flexibility, dynamic balance, and overall good health—in other words, true fitness.

While men are not at the mercy of fashion trends in the same ways that women are, our cultural establishment has expectations for how men should look—strong, confident, and successful. The measures taken in trying to comply with this standard often prevent men from being comfortable, relaxed, and pain-free. More recently our culture has adopted a more muscular, "ripped" look for men, one that focuses on upper-body strength and six-pack abs. Thus we see many men today actively targeting their pecs and abs and working to achieve a certain physical look.

This is a recent phenomenon in the several hundred thousand years of human existence, fueled by a fitness industry that equates "hard body" muscle with attractiveness and health. Not all men try to match this cultural ideal, although many will still admit to feeling somewhat inadequate for not having this idealized physique. They need not worry too much. In the long run all this hard work tends to corrupt the integrated whole of the body's natural design and, sooner or later, usually leads to injury and pain.

At various times in certain cultures women's bodies have been constrained by corsets and girdles that, among other things, served to impair breathing, compress internal organs, and hold a woman's body captive. Free from such restrictive clothing today, even women who pride themselves on being liberated are often

unaware of the compromises they make to their health and well-being when trying
to fit into a culturally imposed standard of beauty. Most women are unaware that
by sucking in their bellies and lifting up their chests while trying to look attractive by a prescribed cultural standard—or alternatively, sinking into a fashionable
collapse—they mimic some of the same constricted conditions to which their
corset-wearing great-grandmothers were subjected.

Americans in a multi-ethnic society are all born into human bodies that share
the same basic design as everyone else. The biggest differences among humans are
cultural, geographic, religious, and economic, but not physical. We speak different
languages and have different traditions, we eat different foods and have different

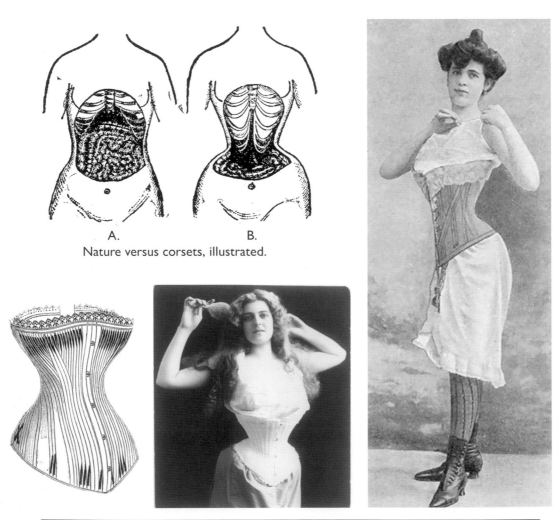

A.   B.
Nature versus corsets, illustrated.

Corsets provide a dramatic example of the compromises women have made to their
health and well-being when trying to fit into culturally imposed standards of beauty.

religious beliefs and practices; but, physically, we are all designed the same way, using the same muscles to move the same bones. Regardless of our inherited size and shape, we all are meant to sit, stand, bend, walk, and even sleep in ways that match the human design. It's the same mechanical system of pulleys and levers that operates inside each individual, regardless of ethnic or racial origin, political or religious affiliation, or inherited body type.

Culture, however, does affect the physical. Any cultural conditioning, such as the messages we learn about how we should look, has the power to take us away from remembering what is natural to us. Even the design of our furniture and the seats in our cars recondition us away from natural use of our bodies. The reason all this matters so much is that this departure from our natural home base often results in chronic pain and poor health.

During photographic research for this book it became startlingly clear that people who are the *in* examples of natural alignment live in far greater numbers in rural areas outside of technologically advanced countries. Many more of the *out* examples—those who've forgotten what it means to be natural—live in modernized, industrialized places. As more and more cultures around the world become influenced by Western movies, fashion trends, music, and pop culture, we face the problem of our entire species forgetting, en masse, how to be naturally human. This raises interesting questions about whether we are evolving or devolving. The growing epidemic of pain and poor overall health makes it all the more urgent that we recognize once and for all what the body's natural alignment is, what we can do to protect it from being lost, and how it can be restored once it has been lost.

In spite of our many technological advances and remarkable medical achievements, many modern-day Americans, whatever our ancestry and through no fault of our own, have not only lost our ability to inhabit natural bodies but also have

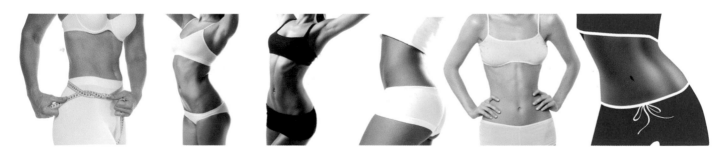

Many modern-day Americans are confused about what good health and fitness really are.

ended up confused about what good health and fitness really are. If we are to be truly healthy and get ourselves back into shape, we must align ourselves, quite literally, with the most basic biomechanical features of our design. The good news is that by examining how some people still inhabit their bodies in a natural way, we can learn to apply universal biomechanical principles to our own bodies to find greater ease and comfort in everything we do.

EACH SPECIES WITH ITS OWN DESIGN

Can you imagine a bird straining its wings from flapping them too hard or a gibbon throwing out its shoulder while swinging from branch to branch? How about a giraffe wrenching its neck reaching for a leaf on a tall tree? It seems unlikely these types of injuries occur, except when an accident happens, such as when a branch breaks or a bird is fooled into thinking a glass window is not there. This is lucky, because no chiropractors or massage therapists, no yoga classes or orthopedic surgeons exist in the wild animal kingdom.

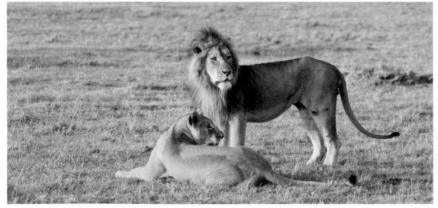
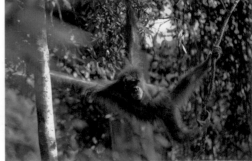
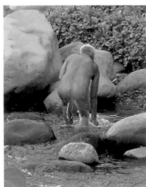
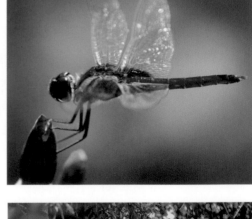
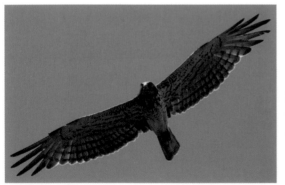

Each species is designed to meet its own unique needs.

Each species comes with its very own biomechanical design that meets its unique needs and defines how it lives. If a bird flaps one wing just a little bit harder than the other one it will be doomed to fly in circles. Survival would become difficult.

HUMANS ADAPT

Humans adjust to demands imposed by influences in our environment. These could be anything from sitting at a computer all day to following examples set by our parents or the culture in which we grew up. Unfortunately, adapting like this often comes with a high price, and we pay for it with a long list of painful consequences. We've somehow fooled ourselves into believing the remedies are far more complicated than they actually are or that we should engage in interventions that often only exacerbate the problems we are trying to fix. In the same way that we have come to understand in recent years that the healthiest food is natural food, as opposed to processed, nutrient-empty food, we must now recognize that the healthiest way to inhabit the body is the natural way, one that honors the design for comfortable, easy movement that is pain-free.

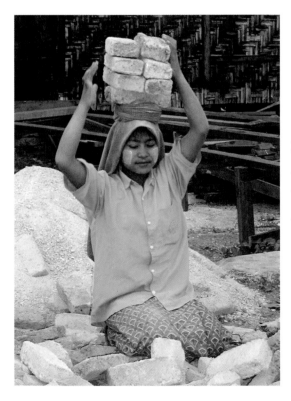

The young woman pictured here carries bricks and rocks for a living. After loading them onto her head, she moves from kneeling to standing with very little effort.

Certain people appear to be prone, in ever-increasing numbers and at younger and younger ages, to throwing out and straining their backs, necks, shoulders, knees, hips, ankles, and wrists while engaging in ordinary everyday activities. Frequently such injuries become a much bigger factor in people's lives than they need to be, and healing is often undercut by well-intentioned but misguided and expensive therapies.

The human body is designed to be remarkably strong and flexible in almost all activities. Many people exclude themselves from this possibility by assuming they are simply too weak, too stiff, or too old to do anything about it. In reality, from the first moment we begin to apply the very same principles used by a small woman carrying rocks on her head, we begin the journey back to our birthright as a human being. While far from a quick fix, we take our first steps toward

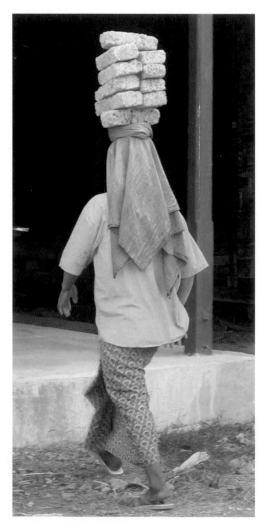

By applying the principles used by a small woman carrying bricks on her head, we can take our first steps toward becoming genuinely stronger and more flexible.

becoming genuinely stronger, more flexible, and more youthful in body. This is a very different process than doing exercises and practicing yoga and other forms of stretching to gain in strength and flexibility.

How can it appear to be so effortless to carry such a heavy load on one's head? The people pictured here are exactly the same species as every one of us, with the same biomechanical design. Most people in technologically developed places would find this a difficult and potentially painful experience, yet these women seem to practically glide through space in spite of the weight of rocks and bricks and fruit bearing down on their heads and spines.

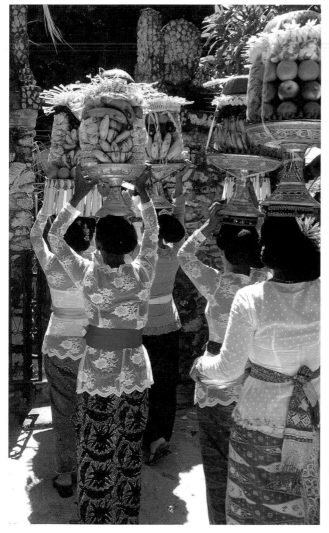

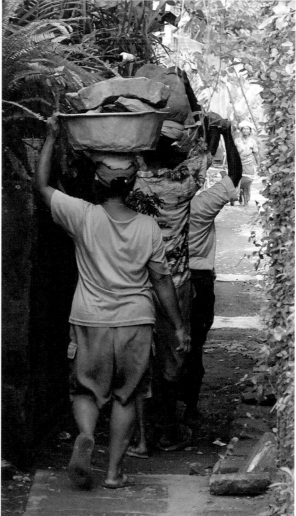

These women seem to glide through space in spite of the weight bearing down on their heads and spines.

Effortless strength

There is no special quality these people possess that makes them able to perform strenuous tasks such as these with general comfort and ease other than the natural human design. The women pictured here have simply maintained a natural ability to inhabit their bodies in keeping with the human design we all discovered as babies and toddlers.

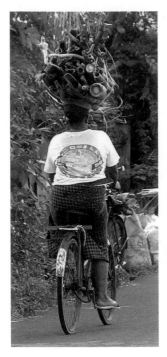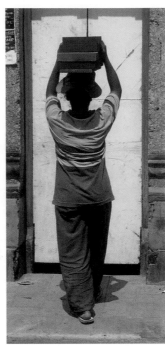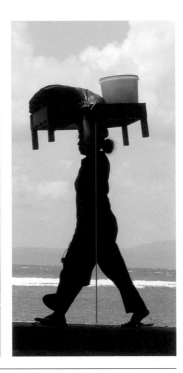

The women pictured here have maintained a natural ability to inhabit their bodies according to the human design.

It is a commonly held notion that the human design is faulty and that we have evolved imperfectly, as if such a thing were even possible. It has been suggested, probably by someone who struggled with back pain, that we became upright too soon—before our spines were up to the task of supporting us in this uniquely human posture.[3] To think of ourselves as innately flawed suggests that we are *apart from,* rather than *a part of,* nature. Such a view ignores the reality of small women carrying astonishingly heavy loads on their heads, sometimes day in and day out for decades, without developing degenerative conditions or pain problems. You and I are unlikely to ever have the need to carry heavy loads on our heads; but with practice almost anyone can overcome many chronic pain issues by learning to rely on the same alignment that makes it possible for these women to carry heavy loads with ease.

This natural human design explains why a middle-aged woman, who appears to be out of shape by our cultural standards, is able to balance a load of wood on her head while easily riding a bicycle. Not only does she give the appearance that this is effortless, for her, and countless other people like her, it *is* effortless.

> A common characteristic of people who live in their bodies in a naturally aligned way is the ease and freedom of their movements, even when they are performing physically challenging tasks.

While the spine is not ageless in a literal sense (obviously, we all wear out sooner or later), the spine's ability to withstand the weight of a heavy head, the forces of gravity, and other stresses that would otherwise accelerate aging is almost assured when it remains aligned along the vertical axis through the decades of a lengthy life. This is true even when we engage in heavy labor over the course of many years, provided that we live by the rules of our design. In fact, being physically active while in a naturally aligned stance only serves to continually reinforce and maintain our basic flexibility and strength and contributes to a level of genuine, easy fitness that can last well into advanced age.

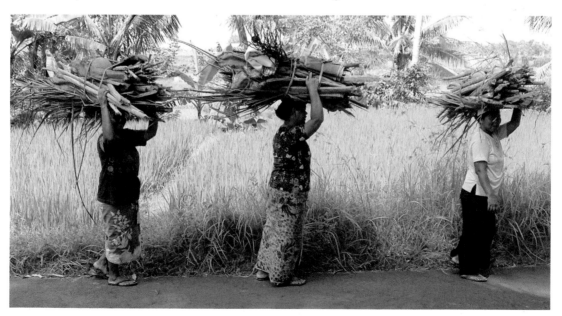

Being physically active while in a naturally aligned stance contributes to genuine fitness that can last well into advanced age.

You may have heard somewhere that people who carry heavy loads on their heads suffer damage to the spine. This is sometimes true, especially in those cases where the bones were not aligned and able to bear the weight through the axis. Indeed, carrying heavy rocks or buckets of water on one's head with misaligned bones is a very bad idea. Carrying heavy loads on the head with aligned bones is often far easier than using one's arms, which is why this is such a common practice in some places.

BABIES AND YOUNG CHILDREN AS TEACHERS OF ALIGNMENT

For those of us who have forgotten how to live in our bodies in a naturally aligned way (which includes almost all of us in technologically advanced places), babies become our teachers. This is because healthy children instinctively teach themselves how to turn over, sit up, crawl, stand, and walk by applying the most basic rules of physics and engineering. If we observe the way babies live in their bodies we can see how a body is intended to work before it develops unnatural habits that are due to physical and emotional trauma as well as living in a culture that misunderstands how our bodies work.

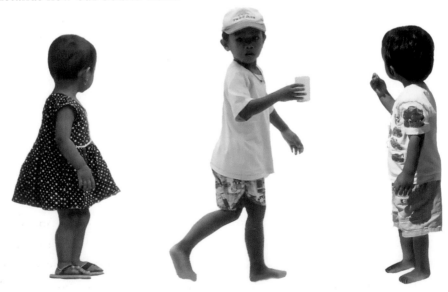

By observing the way babies and young children live in their bodies we can see how the human body is meant to work.

By the time a baby is ready to walk, the work of training the legs to be more than strong enough for full support has been done. For months now the baby has held on to a chair leg or someone's hand and bounced up and down thousands of times. Children learn, through a process of trial and error, to find the positional relationship between leg bones, pelvis, sacrum, rib cage, spine, and skull that best supports the quest to be vertical. Why, then, we might ask, does a child teeter so tentatively while working up the courage to drop Daddy's hand and take that first momentous solo step? Simply put, the child is discovering *balance.*

A baby's greatest challenge in learning how to walk is finding how to balance a very large, heavy head on top of the spine, much like balancing a bowling ball on the end of a stick. Months earlier, when mastering the art of sitting up, the infant completed a shortcut version of this task. In the case of standing, things get a bit more complicated. The mission now is to figure out how to incorporate an anchored pelvis with moving legs in an intricate arrangement of articulating bones and the muscles that move them—all in a very prescribed relationship with one another. Only when this arrangement is in place, stabilized by a powerful core, can the child succeed at delicately balancing a skull on top. For the increasingly rare number of people who are fortunate enough to have never lost this, natural alignment will remain intact throughout their lifetime.

Relaxation is the key to easy balance, and babies are the gurus of how to live in relaxed bodies. Through a process of trial and error, and in a matter of only a few months, they have figured out how to develop the core that anchors them to the world in which they live. This core of stability makes it safe for babies, as well as anyone of any age, to relax. Babies never stop trying to figure out how things work, starting with themselves. Seldom is their incessant playing just a random event, but rather a profoundly motivated drive to understand the details of their design and the world around them.

REMEMBERING WHAT NATURAL LOOKS LIKE

Naturally aligned people have become such a rarity in our part of the world that misalignment has become the new normal. We no longer know what natural looks like. Seldom do we recognize how we, ourselves, and those around us have veered off the axis and adopted a wide assortment of compensating stances, none of which support the body in a natural and, ultimately, healthy way.

In addition to the fairly common problem of misaligned stances, people who

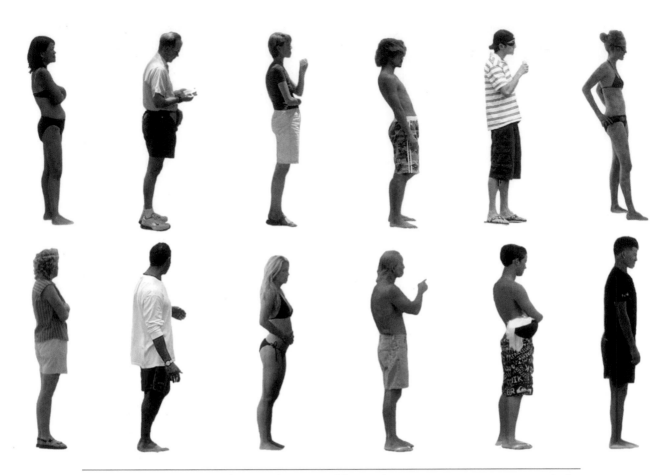

Take a moment to study the people pictured here who, save one, represent a typical cross section of young to middle-aged people found in America today. Only the man on the far right of the second row enjoys the solidly relaxed benefits of deep structural alignment. You can see this in his vertical legs and the straightness of his back. This man is an accomplished surfer, aided by the balance that comes easily to him. Everyone else here is almost certain to struggle in ways that this aligned man does not. They are likely to regularly experience tension and stiffness somewhere in their bodies, perhaps even chronic pain, problems that will only multiply in the years ahead. Even if they are able to find temporary relief by stretching muscles, truly lasting relief will always elude them until they find the support of aligned bones.

have experienced tremendous pain sometimes adopt protective patterns of movement as a way to prevent the possibility of encountering pain. In some instances these protections are based on a remembered fear of pain that was felt long ago. These patterns can lock in deep tensions that compound the original injury. Re-creating some of the earliest movements one would have taught oneself as an infant can reintroduce natural movements that are both safe and therapeutic. Such

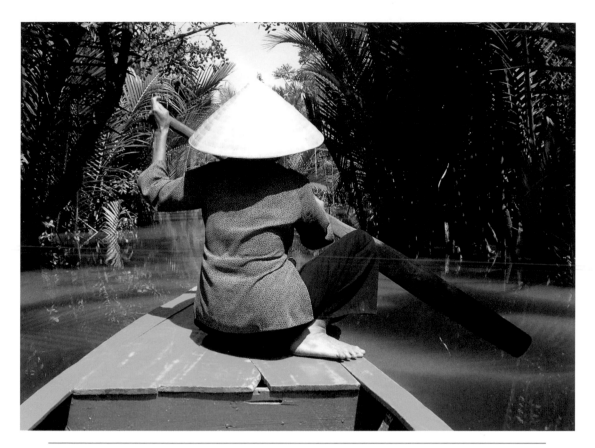

We can acquire strength and flexibility simply by living according to our body's design.

movements retrain the body how to rebuild healthy muscle activity and may even support repair and repatterning of neural pathways. Such an approach appears to be offering promising results for some children and adults with neurodevelopmental problems as well.

Instead of having to work at building strength and flexibility we can acquire and maintain these qualities as natural by-products of living according to our body's design. Rather than having to engage in a persistent regimen of working out to maintain fitness and muscle tone or pursuing stretching programs to relieve tension stored in muscles, we can simply reinforce our natural strength and flexibility in everything we do—walking up stairs, playing sports, bending over to feed the cat, carrying groceries, weeding the garden, sitting at a computer, or paddling a canoe. It is not a matter of what we do but *how* we do it that determines the long-term consequences. Real fitness merges mechanical alignment that is supported by deep core strength. Strength at the core allows everything else to relax.

2

ARCHITECTURE
IN FLESH AND BONE

THE HUMAN DESIGN incorporates many basic principles of engineering and architecture that work to help us fulfill our need for movement as well as to withstand the forces of gravity and other stresses. Our musculoskeletal system operates as a basic system of pulleys (muscles) and levers (bones), not unlike a construction crane. Humans have often borrowed from our own ingenious design to create a variety of mechanical inventions that operate using systems of pulleys and levers. Cranes balance tension and compression in addition to modeling ball-and-socket and hinge joints that allow for efficient bending, rotating, and pivoting of mechanical parts.[1]

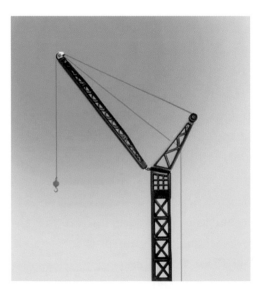

Cranes mimic the human body in the use of a system of pulleys and levers.

We often make the mistake of thinking that muscles and other soft tissue do most of the work of holding us up. This is only true when bones are misaligned and muscles are forced into an exaggerated state of tension to compensate for the lack of correct skeletal alignment. Misunderstanding the role played by bones as the underlying framework of support is behind many bodybuilding and strength training regimens designed to build the muscle strength required to hold us up. In spite of the supporting role that muscles do actually play (except the deep core that we will discuss in the next chapter), the primary function of skeletal muscles is to move bones. For this a muscle must be elastic, able to contract on command, and, free from excess tension, able to relax. This does not mean slackened or stretched out (think of the elastic in your underwear) but part of an interrelated system that stabilizes itself. When bones are placed where they belong they do the lion's share of holding us up; optimally with skeletal muscles toned just so for the supporting role they play and always at the ready to move the bones in less than a moment's notice.

It makes sense that humans, as uniquely upright creatures, would need a design that makes it possible to simultaneously withstand the downward pull of gravity and counterbalance the tensile forces of muscles and connective tissue. The human body shares some features with a structural system called *tensegrity,* which stabilizes itself mechanically by balancing compression and tension forces.[2] Many of the problems that people experience in their bodies result from the fact that the forces of tension and compression are unbalanced, usually with too much reliance on the tensile (muscular) aspects of their design.

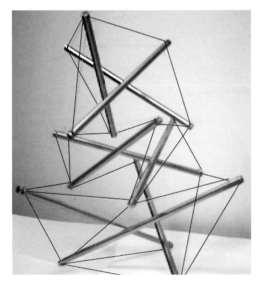

This tensegrity model relies upon equally balanced tension and compression throughout to provide support.

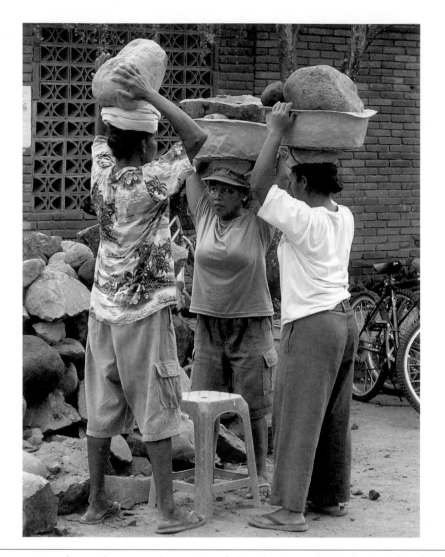

These women rely on the vertical support of their bones to bear the weight of the rocks they carry.

The underlying design that governs if and how the body will move with efficiency depends on the most basic physical laws of gravity. Just as a tall building requires vertical support posts that are strong and perfectly perpendicular to the earth, so do upright *Homo sapiens*.

LET'S HEAR IT FOR THE BONES

Picture a skeleton and it conjures up images of Halloween, graveyards, and archaeological finds. Because the skeleton is what remains of a body after all else has disintegrated, we often think of it as a symbol of death or a gruesome collection of lifeless old bones. If this is how you view the skeleton, think again. Right now there is a living, breathing human skeleton reading these words. The bones that make up your skeleton are dynamically alive, manufacturing blood cells, providing a storehouse for essential nutrients, and playing a part in neural and circulatory pathways. Their complex construction includes an ability to withstand extraordinary compressive forces, yet they are malleable enough to undergo a continuous process of being formed and modified, added to and subtracted from throughout the length of a whole lifetime.

An aligned skeleton sets the stage for the dynamic relationship between aligned bones and elastic muscles that must work together in balance. It is this precise alignment of odd-shaped bones that highlights their compressive features, making

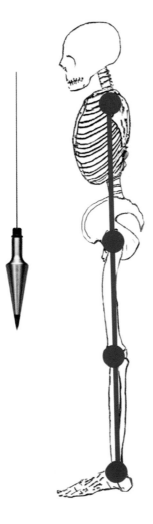

The red line drawn through this skeleton indicates the central axis of gravity that guided each of us when we were learning to become upright. This axis passes through the weight-bearing joints of the ankle, knee, hip, and shoulder, which are stabilized by muscles, tendons, and ligaments that are neither too tight nor too lax.

it possible for some people to carry heavy loads on their heads, with the weight now distributed through bones that align along the vertical axis, or plumb line. With an engaged internal core of muscular support, aligned bones function much like the wall studs and pillars of a house that support the weight of the roof. Bones, however, are alive, malleable, and dynamic in a way that studs and pillars are not.

Far from being the flawed design that some have suggested, the human body is a masterpiece of evolutionary design that incorporates basic rules of physics to the living, moving, upright human structure.

SCAFFOLDING AS FRAMEWORK

The central axis divides the aligned body evenly in every direction. Lines drawn through the weight-bearing joints at their points of articulation, as seen from the front, back, and side, demonstrate the verticality of our uprightness as well as reveal the scaffoldlike framework that applies to our design. Even more reliable and lasting than contrived muscle strength is the enduring, natural strength we have that is bone deep.

Throughout Asia scaffolding is constructed from bamboo, with joints lashed together with twine. It's not difficult to imagine the instability that arises when the vertical foundation posts are askew, causing stresses to be put on the tied-together joints. Ligaments and tendons act to lash joints into place and stabilize them, especially during movement. Perpetual misalignment plays a largely unrecognized role in contributing to much of the current epidemic of osteoarthritis and joint-replacement surgery.

"Bone resembles steel, with the strength for endurance, substance, and stiffness to resist compression and a degree of yielding to sustain shocks. Its resistance to pressure is extraordinary."[3]

Because our bones are oddly shaped and don't conform to pictures we have of other architectural constructions, such as houses, it is easy to miss the precise arrangement these bones must have in relationship to each other, as required by

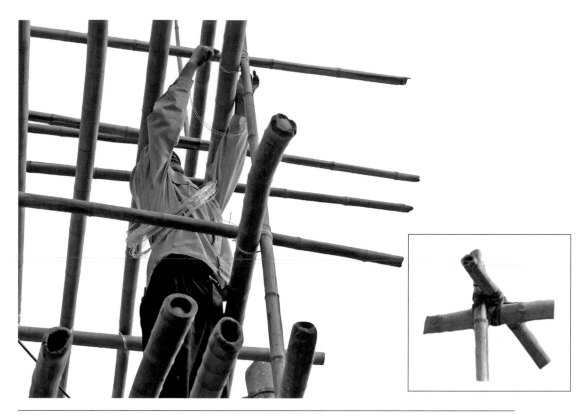

Ligaments and tendons act to lash joints into place in the same way that bamboo scaffolding is lashed together with twine or wire.

the universal human design. Our bones are the framework of support "behind the walls," and, as with wall studs and posts, they must align along the central axis, or plumb line, that all carpenters and builders use as a reference point for verticality. In this way the human skeleton is an architectural wonder of symmetry and functionality.

Babies have no idea, of course, what they are doing when they line up their weight-bearing joints along the central axis. They simply figure out, through intently focusing in a deeply concentrated way in a process of trial and error, that this is how standing works. No one else can ever teach a baby how to sit up, stand, and walk. We can inspire them as role models and encourage them with praise, but all babies must figure out how to do this themselves. Balancing a heavy head on top makes this no small feat.

Our bodies are the houses we live in every day of our lives. We might ask how well the plumbing and wiring can work in a house that is collapsing when compared to a house that is supported by a solid foundation and an aligned interior

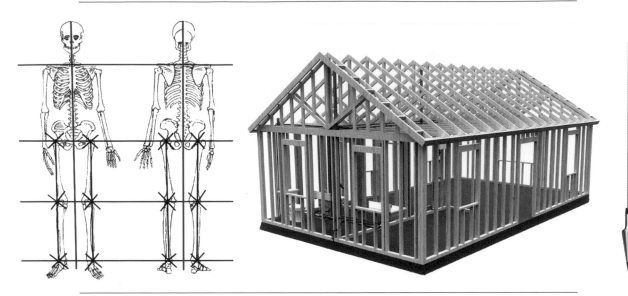

The bones of the human skeleton must align symmetrically along the central axis as the wall studs and posts in the framework of a house must align with the carpenter's plumb line.

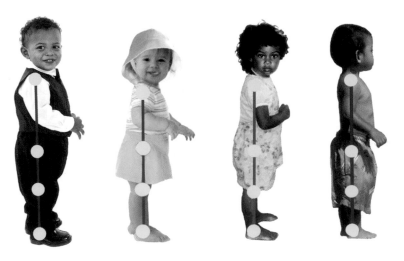

Babies learn to stand by balancing their weight along the central axis.

framework. These are the most basic components that support the body's plumbing (circulatory and digestive systems, etc.) and electrical wiring (nervous system) to be able to function unimpeded. Our cars would never make it around the block if the engine parts were as out of whack as essential, health-supporting parts of our own bodies often are.

Because bodies are able to adapt and work around issues of misalignment, we make the mistake of overlooking what turns out to be the accumulated effect of this over a period of time. Thus we have growing epidemics of many disorders that may, on the surface, seem to have nothing to do with misalignment but which have their basis in organs and other body parts that cannot function optimally when they are chronically compressed and distorted.

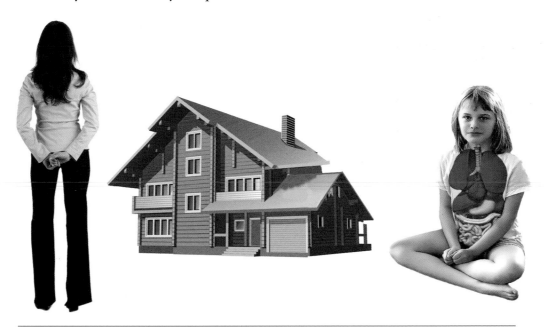

The solidly built house represents the aligned stances exhibited by this woman and young girl, which support healthy functioning of the body's parts.

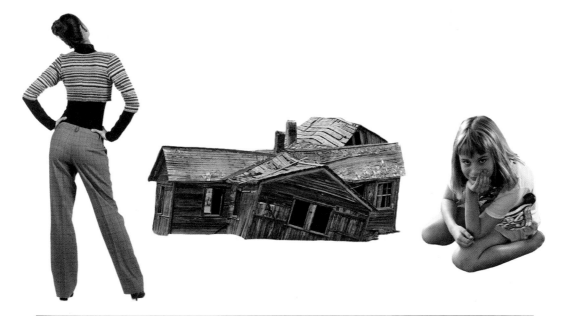

When we continually adopt a misaligned stance over time, our "house" is in danger of collapse along with the distortion and compression of many essential parts.

Being aligned is not about being thin. In the photos shown below the woman in the middle has a larger body type than the others pictured, yet she enjoys the same benefits of being aligned and relaxed. This raises yet more questions about what real fitness might be. While the benefits of a healthy diet and physical activity are obviously important to good health, we overlook the crucial role played by the body's natural alignment.

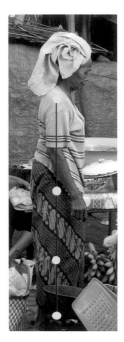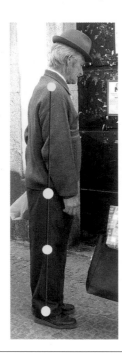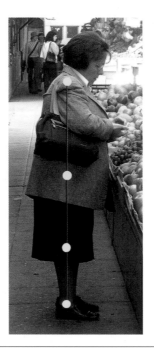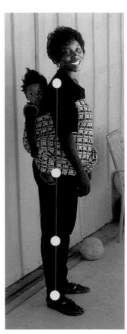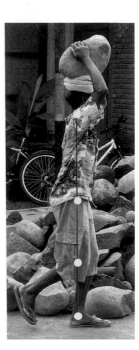

Examples of naturally aligned bodies: note how the weight-bearing joints (indicated by the yellow dots) line up along the central axis.

Characteristics That Naturally Aligned People Share When Standing

- Leg bones form vertical columns of support.
- Central axis divides the entire body almost exactly in half.
- Weight-bearing joints—ankle, knee, hip, and shoulder—line up along the central axis.
- Pelvis and rib cage are in a natural, neutral position.
- Spine is optimally elongated.
- Muscles throughout the body are evenly balanced and elastic.
- Internal organs are positioned naturally and not compressed.
- Body is free from pain and tension.

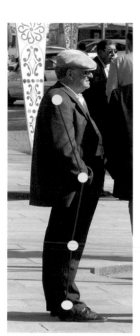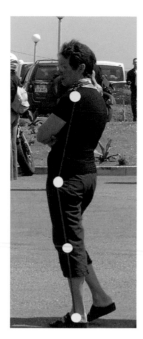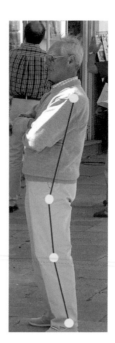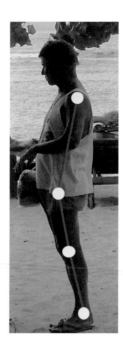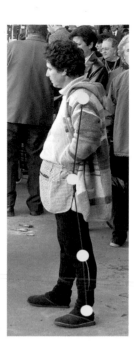

Examples of unnaturally aligned bodies: note how the weight-bearing joints (indicated by the yellow dots) are unstable and under constant stress.

Characteristics That Unnaturally Aligned People Share When Standing
- Leg bones are not vertical and don't offer solid support for the body.
- The skeleton does not organize around the vertical axis.
- Weight-bearing joints are not stacked up, causing compression in the joints.
- Pelvis and rib cage are misplaced.
- Spine is contracted and shortened.
- Muscles throughout the body must be chronically contracted.
- Internal organs are ill positioned, crowded, and compressed.
- The body is subject to chronic tension, pain, and stiffness.

Without the support of aligned legs, the misaligned people shown above must lean the upper body backward in order not to fall forward. This requires tightening a whole host of muscles in the process. It is common for people who stand this way to cross their arms or place them on their hips to relieve the subtle pull of the arms hanging out of the shoulders and stabilize themselves in this position.

THE TRUNK OF THE TREE AND SO MUCH MORE

Alignment of the spine is essential to overall good health and to our being comfortably upright. Each spinal vertebra is precisely shaped to rest on the one below it, separated by a gel-filled cartilaginous disc that cushions bone from rubbing against bone.

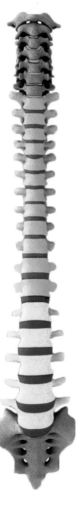

Made up of twenty-four vertebrae and the sacrum on which they sit, the spine is an ingenious construction defined by both stability and mobility.

The vertebral body gives the spinal column the power to absorb and distribute compressive forces, while a complex arrangement of multifaceted joints gives the spine its ability to be fluid and mobile, not rigid. These facet joints enable hydraulic lift and shock-absorbing qualities within the spine when the deep internal core of stability is engaged. All these features, working together, give us the flexible support we need to move with comfort and ease.

The spine has a capacity to rise upward through the vertebral column by engaging with a remarkable phenomenon known as ground reaction force (GRF; see chapter 3 for a more detailed discussion of this). Not only does the spine give support to the torso, it also supports the skull and provides for its multidirectional movements.

The spine's processes serve as anchor points from which the rib cage hangs in a precise arrangement that allows for optimal movement of the diaphragm, the primary muscle of respiration. The spinal cord, as the primary neural pathway for communication to and from the brain, is encased in several layers of membranes called *meninges,* protected within the spinal canal. Optimal functioning of each part depends on the spine maintaining its natural alignment.

SAD DOG, TENSE DOG, HAPPY DOG

Tucking the pelvis disrupts the angle of the legs and takes the foundation out from under the body. Collapse of the skeleton is the result (figure on the left, page 48). This is a "sad dog" stance, because a sad dog tucks its tail between its legs. If this way of inhabiting the body is not corrected, this woman will experience tension, stiffness, and a host of health issues that will grow worse over time.

"Tuck the tail, suck in the belly, lift up the chest, and pull the shoulders back." Sound familiar? Following these instructions creates a "tense dog" posture, because muscular tension and effort are required to hold this stance. While this may seem a preferable alternative to slouching, it comes with its own list of problems that include compression in the spine and joints and chronic tension and pain. If a sad dog represents collapsing the spine, you could say a tense dog collapses the spine in the opposite direction. Neither stance supports an elongated, fully open spine.

Only by aligning the skeleton along the vertical axis do we become "happy dogs," wagging our tails behind us (figure on the right, page 48). Inhabiting the body in this way elongates the spine, maintains natural flexibility, and relies on aligned bones for the basis of our support rather than straining muscles. This posture may appear a little odd or pitched forward if, until now, leaning back with the upper body is how we have perceived "straight." The alignment of joints that stack up along the vertical axis tell the true story of why this is the posture that works.

Wearing a skirt reveals just how much skeletal alignment affects one's appearance, starting with how we wear our clothes. When standing like a sad dog the

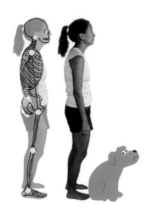 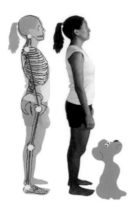 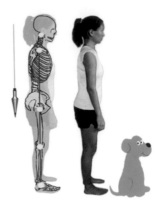

Collapsed Skeleton
"Sad Dog"

Overcorrected
"Tense Dog"

Aligned Skeleton
"Happy Dog"

Comparison of collapsed, overcorrected, and aligned skeletons

fabric of the blouse worn by the woman on the left in the facing photo is bunched up in the front and the back, mirroring the "scrunching" of the spine inside her torso. The hem of her skirt is not straight, but tilted, with the edge of the skirt coming up against the back of her legs.

When adopting the overcorrected tense dog stance, depicted in the middle of the facing picture, this woman's shirt becomes scrunched up in the back but not in the front. This is because she is lengthening through the front of the body at the expense of her now-compressed back. Interestingly, her pelvis is also tipped backward in this position, as evidenced by the tilt of the hem of her skirt.

As shown on the right, when supported by aligned bones in a happy dog stance, this woman's clothes hang like drapery, with a hem that is level. Vertical legs extend down through the middle of the skirt, and the smoothness of her shirt, both in the front and the back, reflects a spine that is elongated and free of compression.

Viewing the photo on page 50, the man's pelvis and sacral platform tilt backward in a typical sad dog stance, causing his upper spine to round or arch forward. This is the beginning of *kyphosis,* often referred to as dowager's hump, a condition that is common among both men and women. People who stand like this often complain of lower back pain. This shortening of the spine becomes all the more pronounced with age, giving way to much more serious collapse as one enters advanced age.

The tense dog stance seen in the woman in the middle is common among

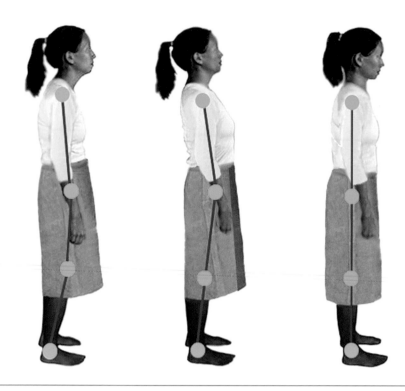

The clothes worn by this woman drape differently depending upon her stance.

some athletes, dancers, yoga practitioners, and people who work out when they engage in these activities with a chest that is lifted up. Exercising from this stance embeds patterns deep into the musculature that often trigger a dependency on stretching and faux flexibility that disappears if the stretching isn't repeated with regularity. Due to widespread misperceptions about good posture, the curves of the spine are commonly represented, even in many medical texts, as having an exaggerated *S* curve, although the spinal curves of healthy toddlers and natural adults are far more gradual than those of a typical "tense dog."

The woman on the right (on page 50) requires little muscular effort to stand upright, because her aligned bones are providing most of the support she needs. Her spine is gradually curved, with the curves existing in the vertebral body of the spine, whereas the spinous processes at the back of the spine tend to be more straight than is commonly thought. This relieves any stress and tension from being exerted on the spinal cord. This woman's vital organs, blood vessels, and neural pathways are all optimally arranged for healthy and efficient functioning. It is rare to find adults in the Western world who still inhabit their bodies with such alignment and relaxed ease.

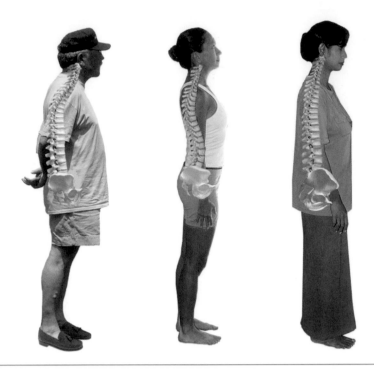

This photo depicts the curvature of the spine in misaligned and aligned stances.

Babies discover how to sit by anchoring the pelvis in the position that supports an upright spine. They do this by figuring out how to rest their weight on the bony runners (*pubis ramus*) that extend forward from each sitz bone (*ischial tuberosity*). Only when the pelvis is planted as a solid foundation can the baby successfully balance a heavy skull on the topmost vertebra (*atlas)* of an elongated spine.

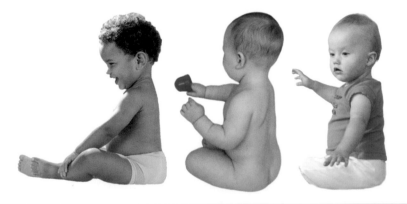

It is easy to see that babies do not use a lot of muscle tension to hold themselves up at this stage. Babies who are developing well and sitting this way also have well-toned core strength that stabilizes the spine in this upright position.

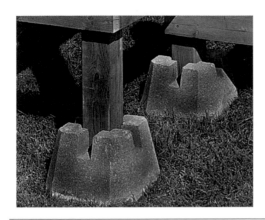
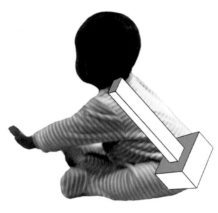

The pelvis serves as the foundation in much the same way that a concrete block is the foundation for a deck post. Babies bend by tipping the pelvis forward and maintaining the lengthened integrity of the spine that neither rounds nor arches but moves as one stable unit. Sitting and bending this way can last a lifetime.

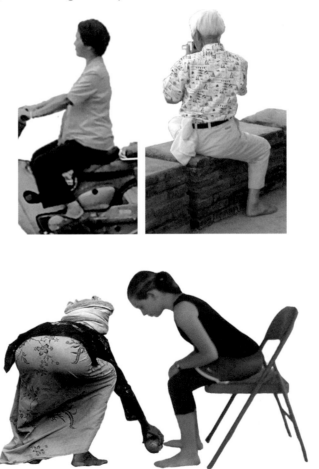

These adults sit and bend with their spines maintained as a stable unit. The 93-year-old woman on the bottom left still bends the way she did as a baby.

TRY IT ON!

Anchor the Pelvis

- Begin by sitting on a chair with a flat surface.
- Place your feet flat on the floor about 6 to 8 inches apart with your knees relaxed open.
- Lean forward slightly and to the left. Place your right hand underneath your right buttock, palm up. Sit down on your hand and wiggle around a bit, feeling the large roundish bone on your hand. This is your *sitz* (or *sit*) bone. These commonly used terms for what is anatomically known as the ischial tuberosity give the mistaken impression that this is where we are meant to sit.

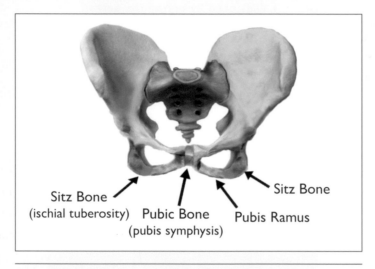

Sitz Bone
(ischial tuberosity)   Pubic Bone
(pubis symphysis)   Pubis Ramus   Sitz Bone

Parts of the pelvis

- Use your fingers to follow the runner (pubis ramus) that extends forward from the sitz bone. This runner follows a line that angles inward toward the pubic bone, or pubis symphysis.
- Draw the front part of the pubis ramus (the *real* sitting bone) behind you, placing it on the chair surface as you slide your hand out from under you. In this position only the front of the sitz bone will be in contact with the surface on which you are sitting.
- Repeat these steps on the left side, beginning by leaning forward and to the right.

Once you have the hang of this you can use the following, more socially convenient, shortcut!

- Lean forward and to the left slightly and "walk" your right sitz bone behind you onto the chair so that your pubic bone is also moving back and down into the seat.
- Repeat on the other side.

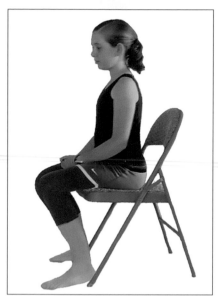

This person is seated on a fully anchored pelvis.

You are now sitting on a fully anchored pelvis. Some people will find that sitting this way causes arching in the lower back, or swayback. We will address this in the steps that follow, but for now, take an inhaling breath and, as you exhale, let your upper body relax and the front of your chest drop down. Sink down into your pelvis. You may feel slightly slouched, for now, but you have also begun to release muscles that, up until now, have been working too hard.

3

THE CORE OF WELL-BEING

WE HEAR A LOT ABOUT core strength and core abs today. Six-pack abs for men and a flat belly for women are held up as the ideal everyone should strive to achieve. We're told core strength is necessary for stabilizing the back, and while this part of the story about abs is true, many misperceptions persist about what real core strength happens to be.

Babies, when given opportunities to develop naturally, begin to build genuine core strength in the earliest months of life. They will put this to use in bringing themselves up to sitting, then crawling, standing, and walking. By the time they are fully upright and walking, they appear to have all the core strength they will ever need. Once lost, however, this deep stabilizing strength can only be regained through a self-directed process of re-creating natural movements that coordinate the dynamic interplay between aligned bones and elastic muscles. This must be done from the ground up and from the inside out.

In the same way that builders never begin constructing a structure at the second floor or try to put the roof on first, we rebuild a healthy body by beginning with a solid foundation. When sitting, this will always be by establishing the pelvic anchor. This is why it is so important for young parents to be informed about how to protect their babies' natural alignment in the first place.

Many popular exercises such as crunches, sit-ups, and the Cat Cow yoga pose, because they shorten the rectus abdominis and reinforce tucking of the tailbone, entrench unhelpful habits in the body and lead us in the wrong direction. Some exercises can be done in ways that are far more beneficial (see part 2), but *only if* the pelvis and rib cage are tethered, at all times, in the proper relationship with each other.

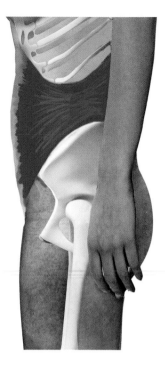

The pelvis and rib cage must be maintained in the proper relationship with each other.

Authentic core strength is not only necessary for stabilizing the spine, protecting the back, and maintaining natural posture, it is also essential to promoting and maintaining a healthy, functioning nervous system. Once this is understood and verified through serious research, many breakthroughs in medicine and health care will follow.

A PARTNERSHIP OF MUSCLES AND BONES

Skeletal muscles are important for many reasons, not the least of which is turning energy into motion by acting as the pulleys in a system of pulleys and levers (bones) that make movement possible. Muscles are the strings that not only animate the body but also engage brain activity so that anything conceived by the brain can be expressed, in nanoseconds, through a muscular response, whether it be bending, reaching, running, speaking, painting, singing, smiling, or scratching one's nose. Without muscles we would be unable to move, respond, or express ourselves at all.

The natural elastic tone of muscle fibers is part of the body's rigging that includes tendons, ligaments, fascial webbing, organs, and skin, all of which, together, lend support to an aligned skeleton. Everything plays its own essential role in relationship to the whole.

Unfortunately, skeletal muscles are often called upon to do work they were never designed to do, such as hold us together when misaligned bones are unable to provide natural support. Muscles function best when attached to aligned bones so that the length and configuration of the muscle fibers are elastic and balanced. If their actions are not balanced and equal, front to back, side to side, we eventually find out about it through the tension, stiffness, and pain that we feel.

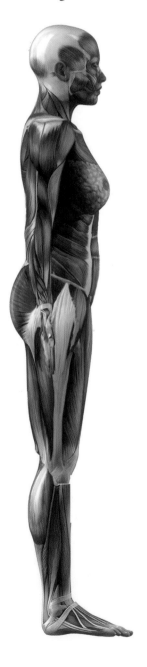

The muscles of the human body, attached to aligned bones for optimal functionality

The key to authentic core strength is the relationship between an anchored pelvis and a forward-rotated rib cage. No muscles are more significant to this neuromuscular interchange than those located in the abdomen, the area of the body's center of gravity—the viscera, the core, our guts. Included among these muscles are the rectus abdominis, internal and external obliques, *transversus abdominis, erector spinae,* and the *psoas* muscles. Not only do these muscles work together to ground the body with the earth, they stabilize the torso and turn on a deep internal combustion engine within the body. The alignment of the bones determines whether these muscles are able to function properly in the first place, while playing a role in determining if the sympathetic or parasympathetic nervous system is dominant at any given time.

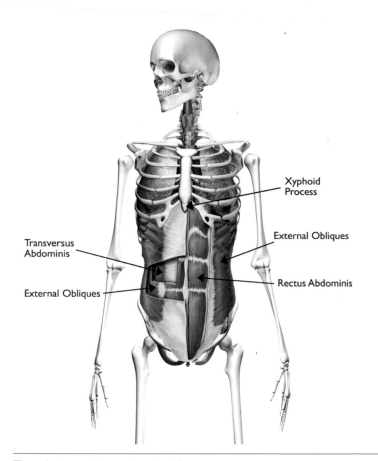

The abdominal muscles that form our core

Strengthening abdominal muscles in an unnatural, artificial way by doing crunches and sit-ups shortens the distance between the pubis symphysis and the sternum, causing the pelvis to tuck, the hamstrings to shorten, the psoas to clench, the diaphragm to be restricted, and, consequently, contraction and compression within the spine.

Think of it this way: in any given moment you are either shortening and compressing your spine or lengthening and opening it. If compression of the spine is a chronic pattern, this will have serious consequences for your overall health as well as defining how you will age. Squeezing the belly through crunches and other front-shortening exercises is still the approach de rigueur that is advised by most health professionals and fitness instructors and practiced by millions of people every day who are sincerely trying their best to get—or stay—healthy.

While it sounds counterintuitive, deep relaxation is at the heart of a strong core. Again, it's about balance: too much unnatural strength in muscles creates continuous tension throughout the body. Even though many muscles play a part in a balanced, healthy core, for our purposes here we are focusing on the four abdominal muscles that form layered sheaths across the middle of the body. Of these four, the core of the core is the deepest. The transversus abdominis muscle is the natural corset of support for the upright body that harnesses vital organs into place. This muscle is weak in most Americans today, especially those people who tuck their butts, exercise regularly by training the abs in a dysfunctional way, or both. We will focus on this muscle in some of the exercises that follow, and it will be important to understand that intended strengthening of this muscle must be coupled with the simultaneous release of unnecessary tensions in the superficial muscles (rectus abdominis) as well.

Maintaining a healthy core must be balanced with letting go of those tensions that interfere with a balanced, homeostatic state. For this we must have the support of aligned bones that makes it possible to surrender the habitual control of holding ourselves together. Nothing is deeper than bone deep. Think of relaxing the bones, and you relax very deeply. Moving your mind into your bones accelerates present awareness, shining a laser beam into the very marrow of presence. In doing this, we make contact with an aspect of ourselves that frequently is buried and goes unnoticed. Such awareness breaks through and short-circuits an unhelpful habit that F. M. Alexander, founder of the Alexander technique, called *end-gaining*, where our focus on the goal continuously supersedes our involvement in the process of reaching that goal. Focusing the mind as deep inside as we can go returns us to *this* moment and encourages us, even as we go about our business, to be in the here and now. It helps to think of bone-deep relaxation as a touchstone we return to as often as we can remember.

The exercises that follow are most effective when done from an aligned, relaxed base. For that you always need the support of an anchored pelvis. There may be many tensions and habits to be overcome in reversing years of misalignment, but being able to let go and release down into the support of an aligned pelvis is always the first step. Give yourself permission to slouch for now. With an anchored pelvis, you won't collapse as much as you expect to, actually, and your body will benefit from having this experience. More active sitting will grow from this base, but the deep relaxation must come first. As you go through the "Try It On!" exercises that follow, set yourself up on an anchored pelvis, move your mind deep into your bones—the skull, ribs, pelvis, arms, and legs, and most especially, the vertebrae of the spine—and with each softly extending exhalation, relax the deepest marrow of your bones.

TRY IT ON!

Rotate Your Rib Cage

Getting Your Back Up

- Sit on a chair with a more or less straight backrest. Your feet are flat on the floor, and your pelvis is anchored. A padded folding chair is ideal for this.
- Imagine you are lifting the middle of your back up onto a little shelf that is just behind you. *Do not* let your pubic bone lift away from the seat as you do this.

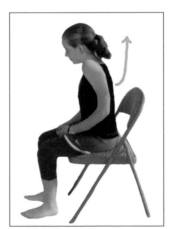

The middle back is lifted as shown here.

- Your shoulders will rise toward your ears as the back of your armpits climb upward. Wiggle your armpits even higher and feel your spine lengthen even more.

- Can you sense your lower back and waist lengthening as muscles deep in your abdomen come to life? Imagine you are receiving a gentle punch in the stomach just under the bottom of the rib cage. Notice how your shoulders roll forward. We'll address that later. For now, don't worry about them. We are only thinking of the lower back and abdomen right now.

Leaning Back

- Repeat this again, this time using the punch coming in under your rib cage to actively lift your back and raise the back of the rib cage high up onto the backrest. *Do not* shift your pelvis. Keep your pubic bone tied to the chair as you lean back from the hips.
- With your back fully supported by the backrest, let your shoulders roll up, around, and back, coming to rest squarely on top of the rib cage.

Exhale and Relax

- Notice the elongation of your spine, particularly your lower back. Using the backrest in this way is like doing self-traction of the spine.

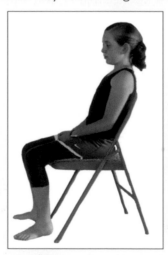

The proper position—
leaning back from the hips,
the spine is elongated, and
the pelvis anchored.

You can also do this exercise while driving your car.

- Set your backrest in a (mostly) upright position.
- If you have a bucket seat that dips in the back, use a small cushion or folded towel to level it out. A wedge-shaped cushion is ideal, as it will elevate your sitz bones.
- Anchor your pelvis.

- Keeping the pubic bone down, lift your back as high up the backrest as possible. You can place a piece of a "sticky" yoga mat behind your back to grab and hold your back high on the backrest.
- Every time you come to a traffic light, repeat this process.

In time, the upper body will also begin to release and open, and you'll be able to sense your neck elongating with greater ease.

FOR EVERY ACTION, AN EQUAL AND OPPOSITE REACTION

We have already seen how easily a relatively small person can carry a heavy load on the head when the vertebrae of the spine are in precise natural alignment. This natural alignment maximizes the body's ability to take part in an energetic exchange with the earth known as ground reaction force (GRF). This is Newton's third law of motion at work, where every action is met with an equal and opposite reaction. If you want a bouncy ball to bounce higher, you will throw it down

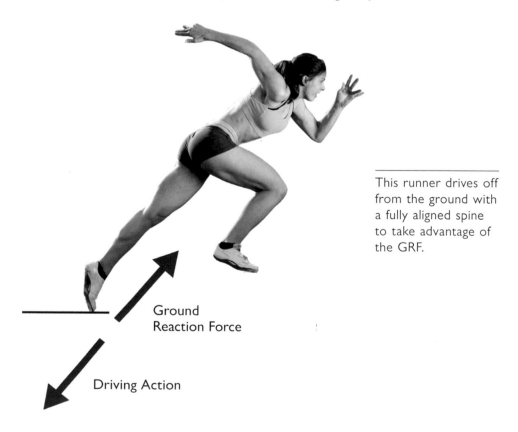

This runner drives off from the ground with a fully aligned spine to take advantage of the GRF.

Ground Reaction Force

Driving Action

harder, causing it to connect more deeply with the earth. If you want to jump high, you have to first drop low while engaging an impulse within the body that pushes off harder against the ground.[1] Someone whose spine is naturally aligned will feel a counterforce rising upward through the spine when jumping up that is similar to carrying a heavy load on the head. Both come from a pelvis that is anchored downward.

Babies learn to engage this GRF beginning in the earliest weeks of life when from their stomachs they are able to push against the surface on which they are lying. This surface acts as the representative of the earth in the same way that a force and counterforce is put into play when a mountain lion gets ready to pounce by first crouching down. The lower the cat crouches, the greater the response through its body.

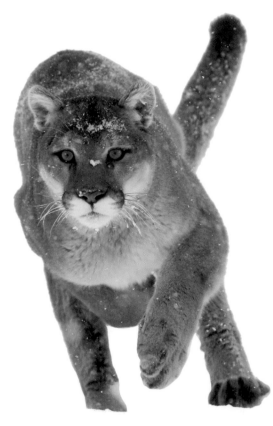

Mountain lion using GRF in pouncing from the ground

Force and counterforce take place naturally in the body when conditions are right. Key to this response is engagement of the transversus abdominis core muscle that serves the dual function of transferring the driving action downward through the pelvis and legs, then up into the torso by stabilizing the spine through which the lift is sent upward. People attempting to carry rocks on their heads would be in a fierce battle with their bodies if they were trying to resist the downward push of the rocks with muscular effort. By stabilizing the core, even if done unknowingly, a person is able to balance internal and external forces, surrendering downward in order to receive upward. This phenomenon is available because of an open, elongated spine through which the weight of the load is distributed. The downward push travels through the body as a driving force and is met with an equal GRF that distributes the weight of the load through the bones. This is matched with an upward rise through the spine. This is why even a small person can move with such ease while carrying a heavy burden on the head.

Babies develop this deep core strength prior to becoming upright. For those who never lose it, this core is never diminished and will support them throughout a lifetime. Not only is this deep core stability the secret of those people who are able to carry heavy things on their heads, it is also the reason some people are able to move into and through old age with elongated spines and flexible joints. (See chapter 7.)

TRY IT ON!

Rotate Your Rib Cage While Experiencing GRF

- Sit with your feet flat on the floor. Begin this exercise as a sad dog, with your tailbone tucked under.
- Gently press your right foot into the floor, and notice the sensations in the muscles of your legs. Can you feel the response all the way up into your hips and buttocks? Notice that nothing much happens above the pelvis.
- Now set yourself up as a happy dog, with your pelvis properly anchored to the chair. Drop your chin slightly toward your chest.
- This time when you press your foot into the floor, notice if you feel the response, at least to some extent, traveling higher in your body.
- Do this one more time, pressing your foot into the floor, but this time simultaneously engage the core transversus abdominis muscle, that gentle punch inward at the bottom of your rib cage that lifts your back up behind you. In other words: the foot goes down and the back goes up.
- Pay close attention to the felt response traveling up from your foot and into your body. Do you sense your sitz bones widening? Do you experience an up-and-down elongation of your spine as the pelvis drops, or roots, downward and your spine lengthens upward through your back and neck?

With practice, you may feel the spine lengthening through the center of your neck, lifting and carrying your head from below without stress or compression of the spine. This is very different from experiencing your head as a heavy load that has to be held up and carried by tension in muscles of the neck and shoulders.

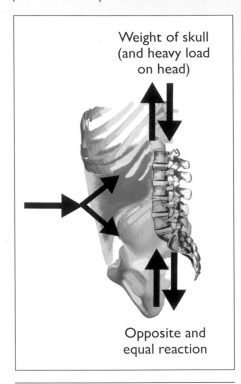

Weight of skull
(and heavy load
on head)

Opposite and
equal reaction

The driving action from below causes the GRF to be transferred up through the spine to lift and carry the weight of the skull.

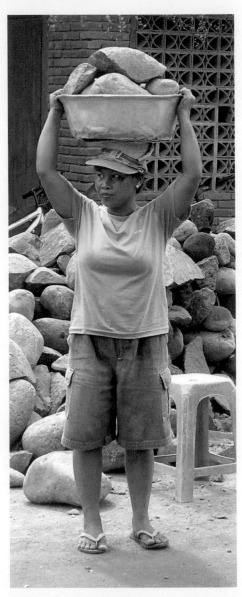

This woman is using GRF, rather than muscle tension, to carry the heavy load of rocks on her head.

Our cultural obsession with having hard-body abs binds up the diaphragm and affects respiration. This creates stress for our entire system. The sympathetic fight-or-flight response is turned on in a low-grade, chronic state. We often don't even notice this is happening, because our regular state of tension is so familiar that it has become our norm. Most of us no longer know what it feels like to be supported by real core abdominals that are naturally elastic—in other words, firm *and* relaxed.

Nowhere is the interplay between GRF and core strength demonstrated more dramatically than in and through the bodies of disabled dancers who perform with great talent and skill while not having the usual benefit of legs. British dancer and actor David Toole was born without legs; Kiera Brinkley was two years old when both her legs were amputated. Unable to rely on the rather lengthy mechanical "levers" that other dancers use to push off from the floor in order to leap and turn and twirl, these two dancers have managed to call forth an innate quality within themselves that is key to their remarkable performances. Perhaps in the same way that someone without sight develops heightened senses of hearing, touch, and smell, David Toole and Kiera Brinkley seem to have drawn into their bodies an extra dose of core engagement with GRF that each one calls on to generate movements that are unexpectedly grounded and powerful. Photographs alone do not capture the fluid movements in the way that they are demonstrated in live performances or in videos. Toole can be seen dancing with the acclaimed United Kingdom dance company Candoco in a remarkable piece at this link: www.youtube.com/watch?v=mLe9ZSwU4aQ. Brinkley can be seen dancing in the following clip: www.youtube.com/watch?v=mgMa1QnBUko.

BREATHING LIFE INTO STRUCTURE

What is it that animates us and brings us to life—makes us so different from an object like a stone or rock? Is it simply a matter of taking in oxygen and expelling carbon dioxide? From a purely mechanistic perspective, this is a large part of what is happening. Oxygen is inhaled and delivered by way of involvement of the lungs, heart, and blood vessels to those parts of the body that need it. Carbon dioxide, a waste product, is then expelled by exhaling. As long as this process is maintained, we are said to be alive.

Breathing is intrinsically connected to energy. In fact, the breath is the fuel that not only feeds every cell but also makes all movement possible. Some people are able to directly experience a subtle energy that is carried by the breath, the life force that animates all living things. In Chinese martial arts it is called *chi* or *qi;* in Japan it is called *ki;* yogis refer to this energy as *prana;* Hawaiians call it *mana.* In all ancient traditions this subtle energy was synonymous with life, the soul, the ineffable enlivening power of the universe. Although we can't remember what it was like to be a newborn baby, it is likely that this pure awareness that babies bring with them into the world is a profoundly physical experience. Imagine their surprise, after being sustained without breath all those months in the womb, to suddenly arrive on dry land and have all the sensations that open within themselves when they begin to breathe.

ONLY ONE WAY TO BREATHE—NATURALLY

There are countless ways to breathe—deep, shallow, smooth, choppy, loud, quiet, soft, hard, free, tight, natural, or unnatural. Breathing exercises, too many to count, have been developed, practically from the beginning of time, to affect the breath for purposes of healing and religious and meditative practices. Managing the breath may have a useful purpose in particular situations, yet only one way of breathing is optimally beneficial for each of us—the most natural, resting breath that requires no control, no manipulation or interference of any kind. Breathing happens, whether or not we are aware of its activity. The multiple benefits of breathing become available when we have the presence of mind to observe its gentle rise and fall and the sensations this generates through the entire body. For many people this can be far easier said than done.

As usual, babies and young children are the role models for how to breathe. Their natural patterns of breathing have not yet been interfered with by a fall off a tricycle, terror in a lightning storm, or the breath holding that comes from humiliation. The accumulation of physical and emotional traumas of early life often embed internal tensions that interrupt and restrict relaxed breathing. Healthy babies are born knowing how to breathe. Soon after birth a baby's diaphragm, along with other respiratory muscles, is already functioning in a natural, elastic way that easily draws oxygen into the lungs through a pistonlike action.

The way babies breathe is soft, easy, and free. Only when they are in distress does the sympathetic nervous system trigger accompanying tensions that interfere with the breath. As soon as a baby recovers equilibrium the breath relaxes again. If the moments of distress become more chronic for some reason, then unhelpful, short-circuited breathing patterns will begin to set in, even at a very early age.

The diaphragm is a large, dome-shaped muscle that serves as the floor of the thoracic cavity, where the heart and lungs are located, and the ceiling of the abdominal cavity, where all the organs of digestion and elimination are located. This muscle must be able to move freely in order for the breath to be natural and free. Loss of elastic movement of the diaphragm through an emphasis on thoracic breathing and unnatural skeletal alignment blocks the free flow of oxygen and energy that is so necessary for comfortable, pain-free living.

A useful visualization for guiding the process of engaging the core abdominals involves a small arrowlike tip at the bottom of the breastbone, or *sternum*. The breastbone is not a bone at all, but a long, flat band of cartilage that runs down the center of the chest, joining the two sides of the rib cage. At the bottom of the sternum is a pointy tip called the *xyphoid process*. We will be referring to this as the *power button*.

This arrow tip can either flip up to the front, in which case the chest pushes forward and lifts upward, or it can aim inward, toward the back of the body. We'll call this action *turning on the power button,* and it will be discussed in detail in the exercise that follows. (You must keep the pelvis anchored while doing this!)

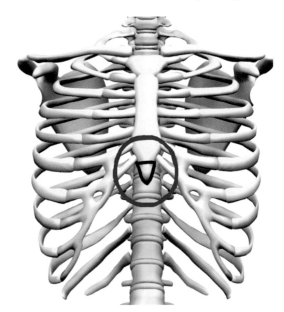

Diagram identifying the location of the xyphoid process

TURNING ON THE POWER BUTTON

Anchoring the pelvis, by itself, is never enough, especially if it causes your back to arch (*lordosis*). The second step, pushing the power button, accomplishes several things at once: (1) it lessens the arching of the lower back, (2) it positions the rib cage along the axis, and (3) it engages the core that stabilizes everything in place. Anchoring the pelvis and turning on the power button are entirely interdependent. If you engage the core without the pelvis being anchored, you'll turn into a sad dog. If you anchor the pelvis without engaging the true core, then you'll turn into a tense dog. Only when both steps are done together will your body respond with the comfort and freedom of movement of a happy dog.

Various images are presented here to give you options to use as well as extra opportunities for the concepts to be clear. More images and ideas, along with additional visualizations, are also included in the chapters that follow.

Assigning landmarks in the body can be very helpful. The pubic bone is a particularly helpful point on the body map when working to maintain the pelvic anchor. It's helpful to think of the pubic bone as always aiming down—or farther down. *Farther down* refers to the direction in which it moves when bending by tipping the pelvis forward. Think of the pelvis not so much as pushing down, as this can cause tension, but extending down. As this happens the two sitz bones will slide away from each other.

Helpful landmarks for the rib cage are the xyphoid process at the bottom of the sternum and a point you pick in the middle of your back, at about the point where a woman would clasp a bra.

TRY IT ON!

Turning On the Power Button

- Sit on a level surface with your feet flat on the floor. Anchor your pelvis.
- Lift the xyphoid process way up in front (don't do this if it hurts your back). Do you notice that your chest puffs up, your back arches and narrows, and muscles in your back and neck tighten? This creates a tense dog situation.
- Turn on the power button by aiming the xyphoid process in toward your back. Again, do not let the pubic bone lift up from the seat. You can even imagine the tip of the xyphoid arrow going right through you and being lifted up onto a high shelf behind you. Your shoulders will roll forward when you do this, but for now simply focus on lengthening and opening the lower back area.

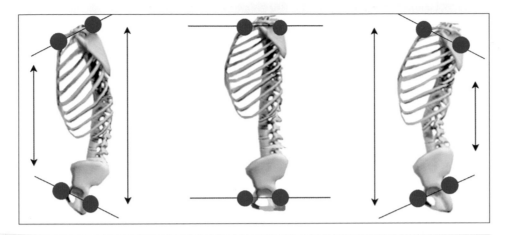

Use these diagrams to help you picture the position of your ribs, pelvis, and spine as you move and perform this exercise.

- As your lower back lifts up behind you, can you feel it becoming longer and wider? Do you feel the engagement of muscles deep in the core of your torso as your xyphoid process moves in and back, lifting the rib cage out of the pelvis? This is more than a little useful, because it engages your core *and* elongates the spine at the same time.

Think of the power button as a way to turn on the core. Soon we'll be placing the shoulders and the head with the help of imaginary wheels and puppet strings.

DIAPHRAGMATIC BREATHING

On inhalation the diaphragm flattens down and outward as it contracts into the abdominal cavity. It creates negative air space in the lungs so that air gets pulled into them, much like the action of a piston in an engine. This action kneads the organs of digestion and elimination; gently pressing and squeezing them with each inhalation and assisting in their efficient functioning. When we are in the habit of breathing just into the upper chest, our organs miss out on this necessary massage. Misalignment of the rib cage and spine can keep us trapped in backward breathing where the inhalation of oxygen is restricted to the more narrow part of the lungs in the upper chest. This engages the sympathetic nervous system and holds the mind and body, to one degree or another, in a heightened state of alert. This prevents us from being able to deeply relax. Chest breathing is common among people who struggle with anxiety, panic attacks, and insomnia.

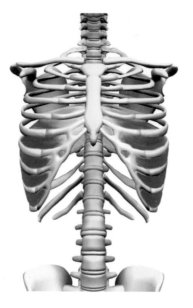

The diaphragm during relaxed, natural exhalation

Diaphragmatic breathing is characterized by the diaphragm drawing oxygen in to the lowest and widest part of the lungs. Deep breathing is often thought of as how much oxygen we can suck into the body on one inhalation, but this approach creates internal tensions that interfere with relaxed breathing. Instead, the inhalation is most efficient when it is soft and quiet and is only deep in terms of its capacity for permeating every cell in the body.

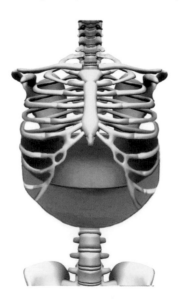

The diaphragm during relaxed, natural inhalation

Just as important, diaphragmatic breathing naturally elongates the spine with a gentle massage, revitalizing the nervous system with each breath. This can be encouraged by getting out of the breath's way so that it can be felt in the back and the sides of the body as well as the front. As the diaphragm relaxes into its dome shape on the exhalation, the parasympathetic nervous system sends a signal throughout the body that all is well and we can rest in a state of calm.

As with every other activity of the body, alignment sets the conditions for optimal efficiency for breathing. When the bones of the skeleton are organized along the vertical axis, the diaphragm is free to rise and fall, like the breath itself, with the same ease and fluidity of a manta ray's undulating winglike fin. As we mindfully witness this process we discover that breathing is not just a mechanism for our survival but also a bridge to the mysteries of life itself—observed and experienced in the joining of physical and nonphysical realities.

SO AS THE PSOAS, SO IS THE PELVIS

One of the most important muscles in the body, as well as one of the least known muscles, is the psoas (pronounced *so-as*). Located deep within the torso, behind the abdominal organs, the psoas is the only muscle that bridges the torso with the legs, passing across the front of the pelvis and hip joint and attaching to the inside of the femur (thigh bone). Merging with the smaller *iliacus* muscle attached at the pelvic rim, together they form the *iliopsoas*.

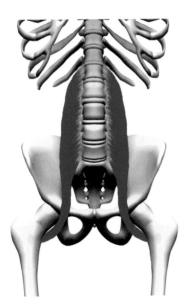

The muscle shown in red is the psoas.

When the skeleton is aligned throughout, the psoas is elastic, able to comfortably perform its multiple roles as hip flexor, guy wire for a dynamic upright spine, and stabilizer of the natural position of the pelvis in relationship to the spine. The psoas and hamstrings at the back of the thighs share a symbiotic relationship. When the pelvis tucks under in a posterior tilt the psoas and hamstrings both shorten, and natural function is corrupted. The clenching of either muscle often translates into back and hip pain as well as being implicated in feelings of anxiety and a fear reflex. Actively stretching this muscle only brings short-term relief and must be repeated regularly unless the underlying misalignment is corrected.

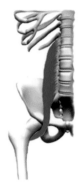 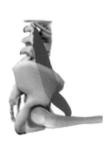 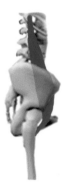 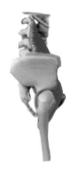

| *Psoas* as guy wire for upright spine | *Psoas* as hip flexor bringing leg toward the body | *Side view of psoas* as guy wire for upright spine | Tucked tailbone causing contraction of psoas |

Views of the psoas and pelvis with the body in various positions

Core strength is *not* synonymous with core tightness. Tightness at the core closes off and prevents the flow of easeful movement, whereas natural strength at the core provides a base of elastic support from which openness, fluidity, and elongation of the spine can occur.

Paradoxically, the psoas, in conjunction with the iliopsoas, can produce different actions, not all of which are natural or helpful. This is possible because this polyarticular muscle (involving more than one joint) responds differently depending on which end is fixed and unmoving.

Among the psoas' important functions is a reciprocal relationship with the diaphragm. A naturally relaxed psoas promotes easy movement of the diaphragm, whereas a tight psoas has just the opposite effect. Conversely, tension in the diaphragm and belly promotes tension in the psoas.

The psoas also plays a key role as part of the fear reflex wherein the body reflexively folds inward on itself, taking up a protective survival mode. This response contracts the psoas as one of the manifestations of fight-or-flight reactions, along with holding the breath, quickening of the heartbeat, and release of adrenaline. Conversely, a chronically contracted psoas, resulting from habitually tucking the butt, can mimic the fear reflex and induce a somewhat constant state of low-level anxiety. People who suffer panic attacks sometimes find relief from symptoms by learning to establish a foundation of aligned bones that allows regular release of the psoas while mindfully observing the relaxed letting-go breath.

A relaxed, elastic psoas is vital to free movement of the pelvis, hips, legs, spine, and diaphragm. It provides balanced support for uprightness through an optimally elongated spine and creates the right conditions for soft, natural breathing that supports parasympathetic nervous system functions (relaxation response).

Natural breathing is not something that can be taught through controlled exercises but something to be rediscovered again and again in each moment. This comes about through first establishing our alignment then continuously turning our attention inward, locating and releasing the tensions that tie us in deep internal knots. Key among these muscles is the psoas. By interfering less with the breath's natural rhythms we come to discover that the body already knows how to breathe without any manipulation or control. Natural alignment of the skeleton cannot be ignored as the place where we must start in creating the conditions necessary for the release of unnecessary tension.

The psoas muscles are important partners in the body's deep core of well-being. Core strength empowers us in a world that is often scary and unreliable. We cannot always rely on events, circumstances, or people to be the way we think we need them to be. What we can count on, however, is the veritable mountain of support to be found beneath our own skin in a dynamic, almost fail-safe interrelationship between bones that are aligned, muscles that are engaged *and* relaxed, and breathing that is natural and conscious.

Tension anywhere in the body acts like bars on a cage that hold the breath captive. Releasing unnecessary tension liberates the breath so that it can be relaxed, free, soft, expansive, and alive.

TRY IT ON!

Will the Real Core Abs Please Stand Up?

- Sit on a chair with your feet flat on the floor and your pelvis anchored.
- Suck in your belly as far as you can and hold it.
- Do you sense your pelvis starting to tuck under? Do you sense tension in your torso and along your spine? Do you notice that you've stopped breathing?

Tightening the rectus abdominis muscles (six-pack abs) at the surface of the belly freezes up the diaphragm, the primary muscles of respiration, which is why you've stopped breathing.

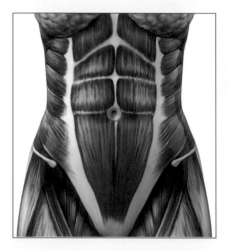

Depiction of the rectus abdominis muscles—six-pack abs

- Now relax and watch the breath return naturally.
- Reestablish your anchored pelvis.
- Pretend to blow out dozens of candles in one continuous stream. Keep blowing until you sense a firming of muscles around your middle.
- Next, cough several times.
- Now, bear down as you would while having a bowel movement.
- Do you sense the same firming around your abdomen in each one of these actions?

While a number of muscles come into play here, each one important in its own way, the one most significant to our purposes is the deepest of the four layers of abdominal muscle, the transversus abdominis, or trans ab, made up of horizontal muscle fibers that wrap around the torso like a cummerbund. This internal corset is the primary stabilizer for the torso and spine.

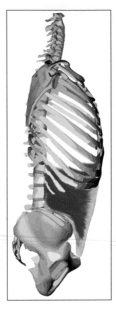

Location of the
transversus abdominis
muscles

- Once again, establish your anchored pelvis.
- Suck in your belly as far as you can one last time, and hold it in.
- Now bear down or engage your trans ab muscle.

Chances are you'll find this much more difficult to do now. This is because the real, authentic core muscles are unable to do their job efficiently when there is excess tension in the more superficial rectus abdominis.

Once again, babies are the role models for how to have healthy abs that are elastic and toned without being tense. Unfortunately, many people have developed unnatural, conditioned patterns in the musculature that cause the lower back to arch excessively (lordosis) when their pelvis is anteriorly rotated (anchored). A retroverted pelvis (tucking the tailbone) is not a viable option for flattening out the arch, because it disrupts the foundation.

The next step in rebuilding our structure will be to learn how our feet must also be solidly anchored to provide the support necessary to carry the weight of our bodies. We will then move on to discuss placing the rib cage in the correct relationship with the pelvis.

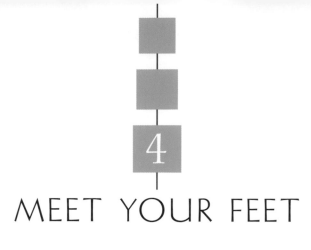

4

MEET YOUR FEET

OUR FEET ARE REMARKABLE structures made up of twenty-six bones each, with thirty-three joints and a complex network of more than one hundred tendons, muscles, and ligaments, not to mention blood vessels and nerves.[1] When we consider that the rest of our bodies are supported on these relatively small platforms, then even large feet can seem small compared to the size of the bodies that stand on them.

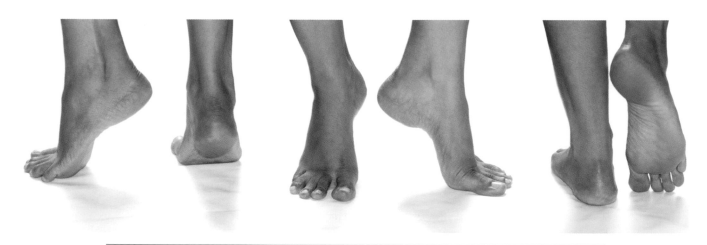

Healthy feet, like the ones pictured here, are supple and strong.

The foot's primary arch (there are several arches) is raised but not rigid or frozen. The lower leg bones, the *tibia* and *fibula,* nestle atop a platform called the *talus,* tethered into place by a collection of ligaments and tendons in a well-secured arrangement. The toes are active participants in the work of the foot, helping to

76

balance weight as well as aiding in pivoting movements and propelling the body forward. The heel is well defined, with the weight of the body aiming through the outside of the foot and heel bone (*calcaneus*).

Our ability to be supported on top of relatively small platforms is due to aligned bones in the feet, as well as throughout the body, that balance the distribution of weight into the feet.

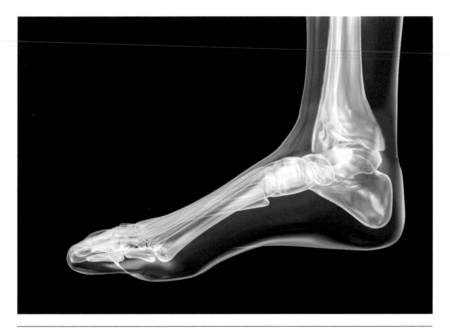

The aligned bones of the foot

Once again, babies and toddlers set the aligned standard for the rest of us. Young children develop strong, vital feet while learning to put weight on them. For many months babies bounce up and down on their legs while holding on to something—building balanced strength and agility in the feet and legs. By the time they are ready to walk on them, their leg bones are accustomed to bearing weight, and their ankles are firmly lashed into place. The toes have had a steady workout through continuous wiggling and having been actively used in crawling and pivoting.

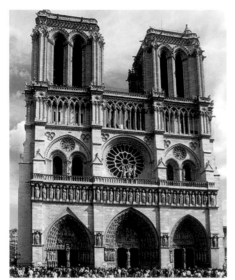
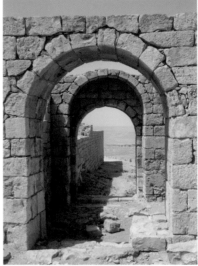
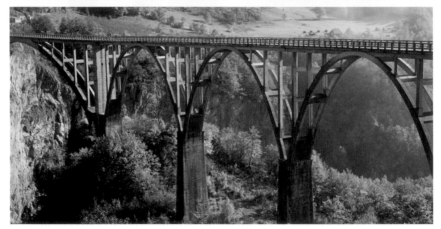

Arches are an extremely effective means of supporting great weight.

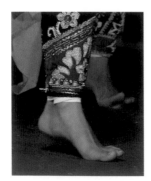
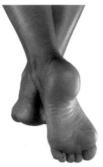
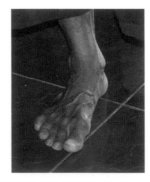
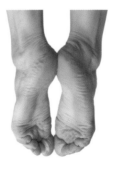

When arches of the feet are well developed they support flexibility and mobility of the feet. The muscles that are required to keep the arches lifted work to help stabilize the ankle and knee joints.

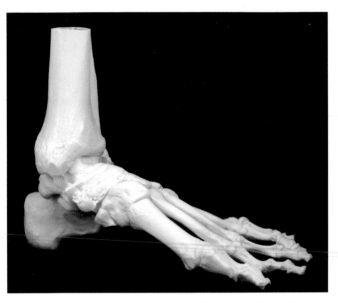
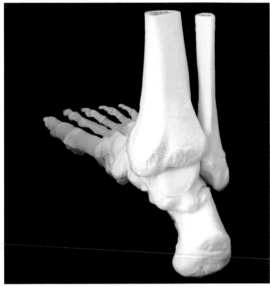

The twenty-six bones in each foot are arranged in a precise and complex relationship with each other that provides a landing pad (the talus) for the lower leg bones (the tibia and fibula). A well-defined and flexible arch is reflected in the height at the top of the foot.

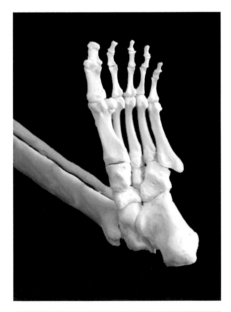

The bones under the ball of the foot are delicate and birdlike and are not designed to carry the weight of the body.

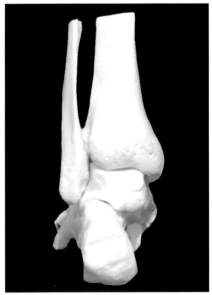

Most of the weight that comes down through the leg bones is sent into the dense, bulky heel bone (calcaneus), which is perfectly designed to catch the weight.

FROM ALIGNED TO MISALIGNED

Misaligned feet create a whole host of problems, not just in the feet themselves but also in the body they are intended to support. Without the support of well-developed arches and stable, secure ankles, problems often occur in the knees, hips, back, shoulders, and even neck. Many people with foot problems find relief when they learn to shift the weight from the balls of the feet onto the heels and to actively use the toes to assist with balance as nature intended.

Some people in the world manage to walk into old age on strong, healthy feet without ever developing modern foot problems such as bunions, hammer toes, heel spurs, and plantar fasciitis. Unfortunately, in the more developed parts of the

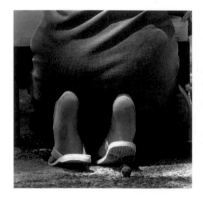 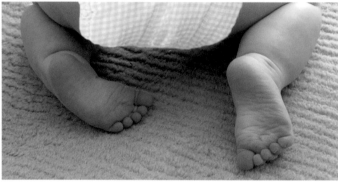 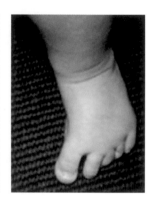

In some populations in the world, especially where people go barefoot much of the time, feet rarely lose the innate qualities of lifted arches and actively working toes. The kidney bean shape evident in babies' feet is often still intact in adults, as well.

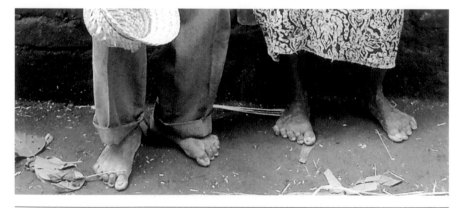

The two pairs of feet pictured here belong to a ninety-year-old man and his eighty-six-year-old wife. They work barefoot every day in the rice paddy behind their home and have rarely worn shoes during their lives. Their feet are remarkable in how much they still resemble the feet of young children.

world these types of problems are not uncommon. The cause is not lost though, and we will explore, later in this chapter, an exercise that can be used to realign the bones of the feet and repair the damage caused by habitual misalignment and poor posture.

The alignment of the feet is reflected in the relationship of the legs and pelvis and vice versa. The man on the left in the bottom photo has feet that still support him the same way they did when he was a child. The plaid print of his sarong graphically demonstrates the straightness of legs that serve as pillars of support

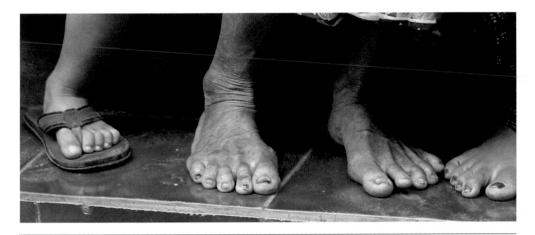

The pair of feet pictured in the middle of this photograph have helped this woman carry river rocks on her head, which she did for several decades. They now help her assist with the daily care of her great-grandson, whose feet are pictured next to hers. At one hundred and three years old, these feet continue to be healthy, strong, and flexible.

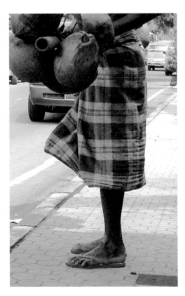 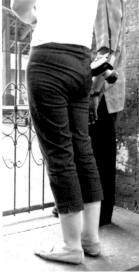

A comparison of how these two people are standing highlights what happens when we do not align our bodies and our feet.

and distribute the weight of his body through active, aligned feet. This is not the case for the woman on the right (on page 83), whose pelvis is severely tucked under, causing her legs to angle diagonally out from under her. This is a far more common way of standing in our society, than that of the man on the left. The woman's ankles are pronated, disrupting support for an already-collapsing structure above. The weight of her body lands very differently from the way the weight lands on the man's feet. Although she is only in her late thirties, it is not surprising that she is complaining of pain in her back and her knees, while the man, who is seventy-eight years old, reports no pain in his body.

Something as seemingly insignificant as the kinds of shoes one wears or various stresses to the feet set the stage, quite literally, for whether the body that is carried above is able to participate in a dynamic exchange with the earth. Thus begins for many people a long, slow descent from being upright and vital to having lost essential support from the bottom up.

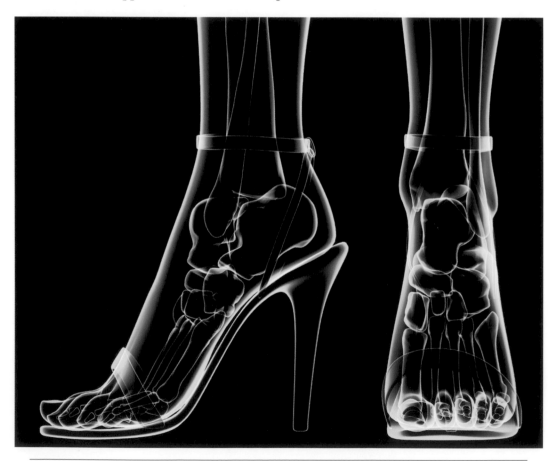

Disruption of the natural arrangement of the bones of the feet makes it virtually impossible for the body above to be aligned.

Collapsed Arches

Collapsed arches contribute to a long list of problems that can develop as a result of faulty foundational support. In most cases the knees are medially rotated (turned inward), causing the ankle to roll in and the leg bones to aim off the top of the ankle platform. This causes a shear force upon the ankle joint, making it unstable and prone to being twisted and sprained. The knee and hip joints are also vulnerable without solid, aligned support from below. Muscles of the leg are torqued and misshapen, with some being chronically shortened, while others are chronically stretched out.

Many feet tend to function more like flippers that slap along the ground when they walk. Without arches they are unable to provide the body with the shock-absorbing qualities that healthy feet are designed to do. The toes are uninvolved and are of little help in walking. Instead of the weight of the body landing on the heel and being distributed in a balanced way throughout the foot, the weight comes down on the insides of the feet with a somewhat deadening effect that disrupts the ability of the whole body to connect by way of GRF with the earth.

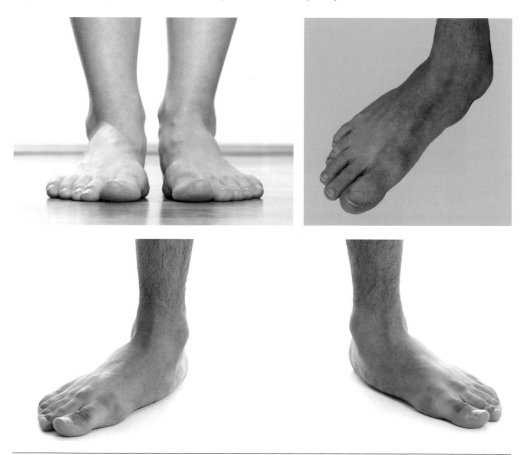

Examples of "flipper" feet with fallen arches

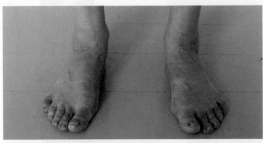

Be sure not to lift your toes or the ball of your foot.

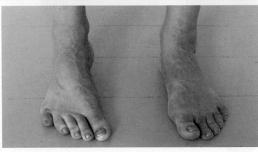

The heel moves to the center as you rotate your knee to the right, changing the shape of your foot.

- Bring the right heel onto the floor and let your weight come to rest squarely on the heel. It may feel like your weight is on the outside of the foot. Compare the appearance of the left and right feet and take a moment to reflect on the differences in how your two legs feel. Which leg feels more solid? Which leg feels more actively engaged?

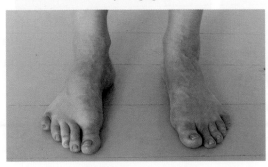

Your heel is now firmly on the ground, with the weight more to the outside of the heel.

- Repeat on the left side.

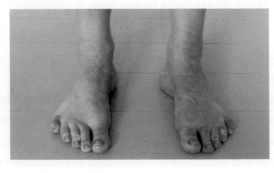

Now both feet are solidly planted.

Frequent and regular practice of the steps outlined above can have dramatic results and provide lasting relief from many of the complications of a failure to maintain the natural alignment of the foot and its stable connection with the ground. Bending often and bending well (see page 246) strengthens the muscles that lift the arches and stabilize the ankles.

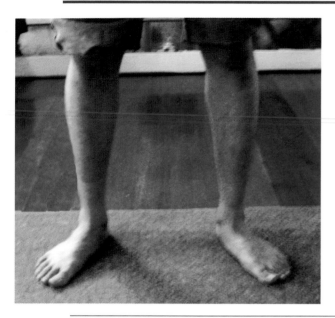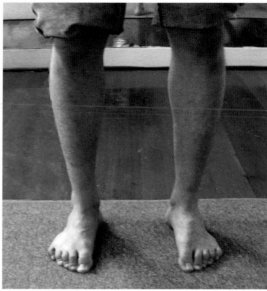

These feet belong to a young man who found relief from persistent back pain when he reshaped his feet. As with the bunion photographs discussed previously, these were taken moments apart and show a striking change. As long as this man continues to tuck his heels, his legs will be solid, his knees stable, his toes active, his arches lifted, and the weight of his body will land on the outside of his heels. Although far from a quick fix, as these steps must be practiced repeatedly for muscles to reprogram and begin to hold up the arches, this represents a much more meaningful and proactive improvement over simply wearing expensive orthotic inserts, which often do not address the underlying cause of the problem.

Healthy feet engage with the ground on which they stand. They serve the body for many decades, and their strength, flexibility, and alignment is reflected in the health of the body that stands above them.

Lately there has been a great deal of interest in a new trend in footwear called "barefoot technology." Several brands of shoe have been designed with the intention of protecting the sole of the foot while providing the benefits inherent in running with bare feet. Some of these shoes fit the foot much like a glove, with individual compartments for each toe. Other shoes have been designed with a

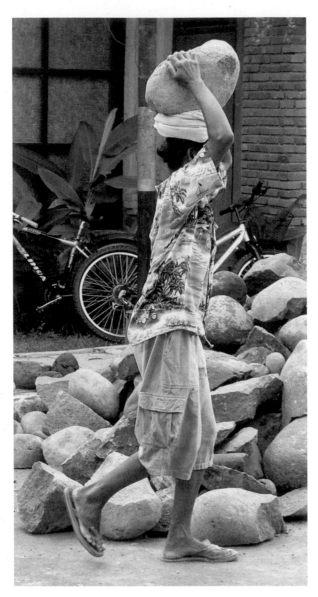

This woman's feet and legs are the transportation system for her entire body and support the pelvis, spine, rib cage, and skull in a balanced relationship that allows her to carry rocks like this all day, every day (*even* on pavement).

rocker bottom, ostensibly to mimic the feet of Masai tribesmen in Africa. While some people feel that these various shoes have been beneficial to them, others have complained of joint pain and other injuries as a result of using them. It is important to remember that a shoe alone is unlikely to resolve underlying structural problems. In the long run it is better to learn the rules for inhabiting the body as naturally as possible while wearing shoes that are soft, rather than rigid, and that provide ample space for the toes to remain active within the shoe. When running the knees should track to the outside, while the body is led forward by the back of the rib cage and back of the head rising up and forward—not by a lifted chest.

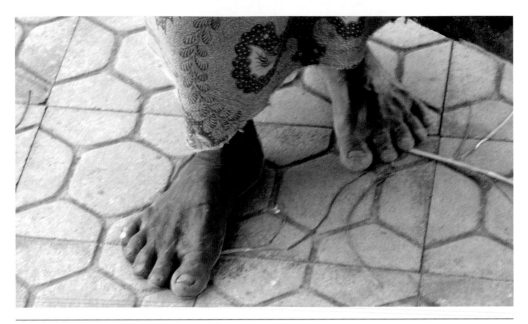

The secret to this woman's success is good arch support—not the kind that comes with expensive sports shoes but her very own built-in arches.

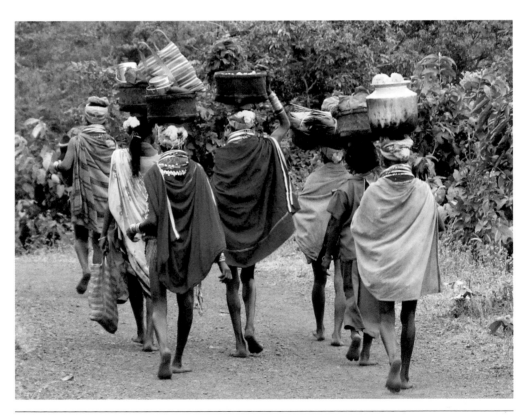

These people are all carrying heavy loads on their heads. A close look at their bare feet shows them to have the kidney bean shape characteristic of all healthy, natural feet. The weight comes down onto a solid pillar with weight distributed through active, supple feet.

5

WHEELS, BELLS,
AND PUPPET STRINGS

ALTHOUGH THE SKELETON is a complex structure made up of 206 bones, it can be more broadly thought of as consisting of three primary structures—pelvis, rib cage, and skull—plus one spine and two arms, legs, hands, and feet. The pelvis, rib cage, and skull all relate to each other by way of the spine to which each is connected. We run into trouble when we have patterns of movement and ways of inhabiting the body that disrupt the natural relationship among these bony structures.

Changing deeply embedded habits is challenging for anyone. The use of imagery is a handy way to understand how the bony structures are intended to relate to each other as well as providing a straightforward technique for learning how to bring the body back to its natural home base. The images presented in this chapter are designed to offer yet another way of understanding the details of what natural skeletal alignment looks like as well as provide you with useful tools for guiding yourself through the task of making changes that can work in a lasting way. There are any number of images that could be used to do this, so feel free to think up your own—provided they accomplish the same results, of course.

THREE WHEELS OF ALIGNMENT

The skull, rib cage, and pelvis all share a basic roundness to their shape. Imagining these round shapes as wheels that can turn backward or forward, independent of each other, provides a useful map for analyzing the alignment of any body.

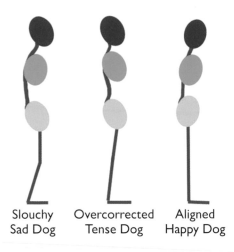

Slouchy   Overcorrected   Aligned
Sad Dog   Tense Dog   Happy Dog

By assigning oval shapes to these three wheels, it becomes easy to see in which direction each wheel is turning.

The direction the wheels are turning defines whether a skeleton is able to support the body with authentic strength and enduring ease of movement. In other words—is the pelvis tucked under or rotating forward? Is the rib cage rotating backward, requiring that it be held up with tension, or does it hang naturally from the processes of the spine? There are numerous variations and degrees of misaligned collapse, but only one way of being aligned.

We can see in the sad dog stance that the pelvic wheel is rotating backward. This takes the legs out from under the body. The chest wheel sinks down and the head wheel rolls back.

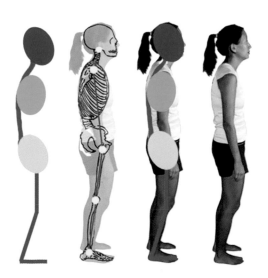

Sad dog stance with the head and pelvis wheels rotated back and the chest wheel rotated forward.

There are many variations of slouching, yet they all share the same basic elements. Slouching starts when the pelvic wheel rotates backward. This takes the legs out from under the body, causing them to be weak and unable to adequately support the body above them. The rib cage sinks down into the pelvis, causing shortening and compression throughout the torso. The neck and chin are thrust forward, compressing the cervical spine as the head tips back. Two wheels backward and one wheel forward is the signature arrangement of slouching.

The most common instruction to counteract slouching, as previously mentioned, is to tuck the butt, suck in the belly, lift the chest, and pull the shoulders back. These instructions are burned into almost everyone's mind as the correct way to achieve "good posture," yet following these instructions causes a tense dog stance with all three wheels rotating backward.

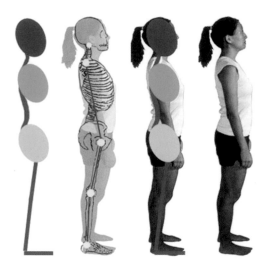

The usual tendency to counteract slouching is to lift the front of the body upward like a soldier standing at attention. This clearly causes each of the three wheels to roll backward in a tense dog stance.

At first glance the front of the body looks more open than the slouching stance, but the back of the body is shortened and compressed. The weight of the head and upper body bears down and puts stress on the weight-bearing joints below. The legs are set at a diagonal angle, not directly under the body, and the lifting of the chest often causes the knees to lock. Would you want to live in a pole house supported by foundation poles that are not aligned along the vertical axis?

It is interesting that the aligned stance, which is the most natural, is the one that can appear to be a little odd if you have been conditioned to think the above way of standing represents good posture. In the happy dog stance we see all three wheels turning forward. The legs are lined up along the axis, able to provide the kind of support that is needed for the body above them. The front and the back of the body are both long and open, in a balanced kind of way that prevents the distortion or compression of the spine, organs, muscles, and all other soft tissue. Veins and arteries are open channels for the circulation of oxygenated blood throughout the body.

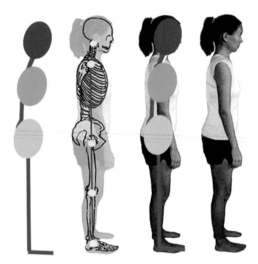

The aligned, happy dog, stance can look different, strange even, if you have always believed that the tense dog stance is what good posture looks like.

Everyone's individual posture fits somewhere on this wheel map. Some actors are particularly talented in their ability to portray a variety of characters, in part because of their own natural alignment, which gives them a full range of options and the freedom of movement to bring a variety of characters to life. Character actors are sometimes people who, because of chronic postural misalignment, are stuck in a particular way of inhabiting the body. When this is the case they have fewer options and tend to play the same types of roles over and over again.

No matter how your own wheels are presently arranged, the basic formula for reclaiming your home base of natural alignment is essentially the same for everyone: turning all three wheels forward, one on top of the other. This is the action that organizes the entire skeleton around the vertical axis and that elongates the spine up through the back.

TURNING THE PELVIC WHEEL

We already know that the biggest culprit of collapse is a backward-tilting pelvis that is unable to support a naturally upright spine. So we can see very clearly that the first step to resolving this collapse is to turn the pelvic wheel forward.

When the pelvis is habitually tucked under, the muscles around the hips, thighs, buttocks, and abdomen are all conditioned to work in an unnatural way. This greatly limits the various options for natural, free movement. Doing specific exercises may bring some relief from tension or discomfort, but the relief is only temporary until the pelvis is anchored in its natural position. Maintaining this pelvic anchor while standing, bending, walking, and sitting retrains the body to take on more helpful, natural habits.

The image of the pelvis as a bowl is one that is often used to describe the pelvis. *Pelvis* means "basin" in Latin and, while there are obvious similarities, this view of the pelvis can be misleading. It may be more useful to picture the pelvic bowl tipped all the way onto its side. The bottom rim of the bowl illustrates the way the pubis symphysis (pubic bone) aims downward and the sitz bones slide out behind.

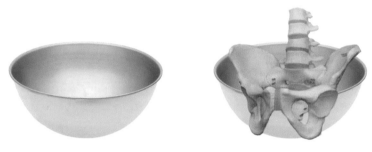

Backward-rotated, "tucked" pelvis

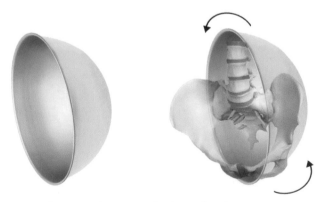

Anteriorly rotated, aligned pelvis

The properly aligned pelvis may be viewed as a bowl tipped on its side.

Natural movement is initiated from the core, with the upper pelvic rim leading the way and the pubic bone aiming down. Any contents of the pelvic bowl would be poured out the front anytime bending forward occurred. If you feel your back arching when doing this, remember this is only the first step. The next step will stabilize the relationship between the pelvis and the rib cage. If doing this hurts, stop for now. You can try again after you've learned the next step—how to rotate your rib cage.

TURNING THE RIB CAGE WHEEL

It can be hard to believe that tension in the abs has to be relaxed in order to strengthen the deeper core, especially when almost every cultural message tells us otherwise. Poor postural habits, such as a tucked butt, interfere with the deeper core muscles' ability to engage. Overdevelopment and contraction of the more superficial rectus abdominis muscles is like a glue that binds the rib cage and pelvis together and restricts natural movement. Releasing tension in the belly loosens the glue and allows the pelvis and rib cage to move independent of each other.

Optimal length of the spine depends on the rib cage wheel turning forward. Sucking in the belly or lifting the chest, both actions that so many people think they should be doing, actually shortens, rather than lengthens the spine.

TRY IT ON!

Turning Your Wheels

- Sit on a chair with your feet flat on the floor.
- This time, as you anchor your pelvis, imagine your pelvis as a bowl tipping onto its side. If the bowl were filled with water, all of it would pour out the front of the bowl.

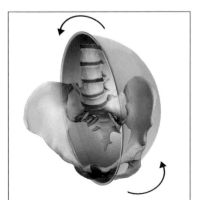

The pelvic bowl
should tilt forward.

- Now roll your weight back and forth on the bottom of the pelvis, as the pubic bone lifts away from the seat, then aims down again.
- Do this a few more times and notice if your rib cage also moves with the shifting pelvis. Chances are, as your tailbone tucks under, your chest collapses and your back rounds, and as the pubic bone rolls down into the seat the chest lifts and the back arches. *Stop* if this causes you any pain.
- Anchor your pelvis again, not letting it move as you rotate your rib cage wheel in the two directions pictured below, isolating the movement from a solidly anchored pelvis. (Use your power button to stabilize the position of the pelvis if your pubic bone wants to automatically lift off the chair as you do this.)

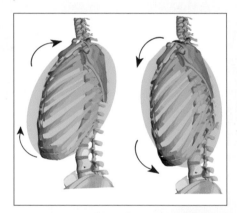

Tilt your rib cage backward and forward from a solidly anchored pelvis.

- Do this slowly and notice the sensations you experience as your rib cage wheel rolls back and the chest lifts (back arches and shortens) and then as the rib cage wheel rolls forward and the sternum moves toward your back (back lengthens and widens).

TURNING THE HEAD WHEEL

The weight of an average adult head is equivalent to that of a standard bowling ball. This means that, with or without a pile of rocks on our heads, we are already carrying a heavy load on top of our spines. Imagine how hard your neck muscles must work to support your head when it is not poised as it should be on top of the spine.

Most people, when asked where the head and spine meet, will point to the base of the skull, the *occiput*. Yet when asked to balance a ball on a stick they place the stick at the center of the ball, not at the edge. Exactly the same principle applies to a head that is designed to balance delicately on top of the spine.

If you draw an imaginary line from the tip of your nose out through the back of your head and another line between your ears, the point behind your nose where these two lines intersect is the approximate place where your skull balances on top of the spine. The two uppermost cervical vertebrae, the atlas and the axis, work together in an ingenious way to allow tension-free, relaxed, and easy rotational movements of the head and neck such as nodding the head *yes* and shaking the head *no*.

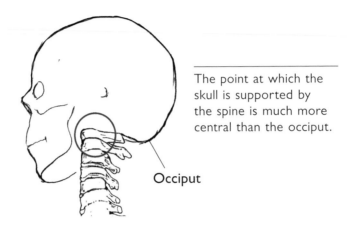

The point at which the skull is supported by the spine is much more central than the occiput.

Occiput

When all three wheels are turning in the forward direction, the spine is optimally elongated along the back. At the base of the neck the spine shifts so as to rise up directly beneath the middle of the skull. In fact, this rising spine is designed to support the skull from below instead of the weight of the skull pressing down onto the spine, which is the cause of many people's neck problems. If you've ever balanced the end of a broom on the tip of your finger, you can now imagine the top of your spine acting in the same way as the finger, while the skull balances delicately like the broom, lifted from below. Many people find great relief from neck and shoulder strain simply by knowing and experiencing the relationship between the spine and skull this way.

The head can be a heavy burden we struggle to carry around all day. When the chin leads out in front (figure on right, page 100) it sends all the weight into the back of the skull, jamming the head down onto the *atlanto-occipital* joint and collapsing the neck. This forces neck muscles to strain and can contribute to headaches, neck and shoulder strain, and compression elsewhere in the spine. Dropping

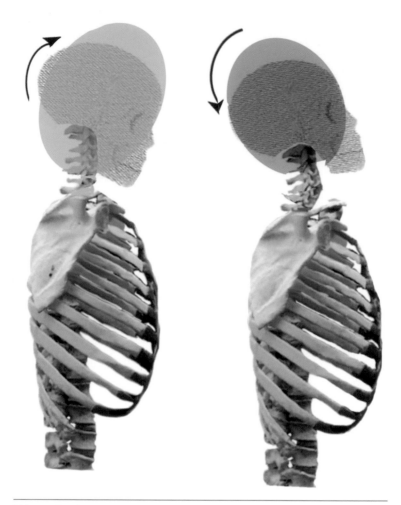

Tilting the head back collapses the neck and results in misalignment of the spine.

the head back plays a big part, along with a tucked pelvis, in the development of kyphosis, or dowager's hump, as one ages.

As you read this lift your chin, then gently drop it toward your chest. Do this slowly a few more times, just far enough to sense how your cervical spine (neck) lengthens in the back when your chin is dropped and shortens when you lift your chin. The weight shifts forward into the front portion of the cranium as the chin drops slightly toward the chest. Many people find this a difficult concept to accept, because we've been conditioned by cultural messages to believe the head belongs in the backward-tipping position. "Chin up," we're told from an early age.

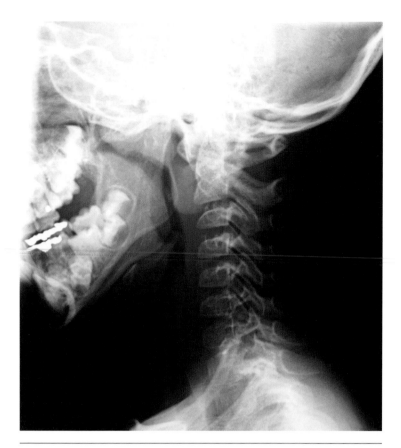

This x-ray shows a properly aligned spine with the head tilted gently forward, elongating the neck.

When it comes to the ways in which the body is a metaphor for how we live our lives, this may be one instance where holding your head up high is not helpful. Not only does this cause the chest and chin to lift, with all the resulting tensions, but such a stance can convey a false impression of arrogance or lack of humility.

It takes practice and patience to get used to the new feelings that come with letting the head balance on top of the spine. Learning to relax unnecessary tension in the belly helps relax the neck, which in turn frees the head and releases tension at the atlanto-occipital joint where the spine and skull meet.

RINGING THE BELLS OF ALIGNMENT

Another useful way to picture the three primary bony structures of the skeleton is to imagine them as bells. This is a simplified version of the three wheels analogy that doesn't include the spine but offers another way to envision the positioning of the bones.

In this case the pelvis, rib cage, and head are imagined to be three large bells, much like those found in the bell tower of a church. Of course, if these were real bells, all the clappers would not remain unmoving in the middle of the bell. For our purposes here, however, they have been left suspended in the center in order to better demonstrate the angle of distortion of the spine's trajectory.

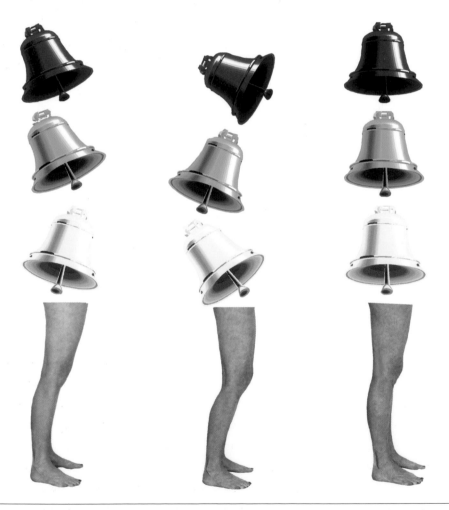

The bells representing the head, rib cage, and pelvis tilt to demonstrate how the rotation of these body parts can affect the body's alignment.

PELVIC FLOOR HAMMOCKS

It can be difficult to believe that the floor of the pelvis should be relaxed, especially when many exercise programs and cultural messages tell us otherwise. The muscles of the pelvic floor become chronically contracted when we tuck the tailbone under and suck in the belly. Suck and tuck. Tucking the tail under is what a dog does when it is cowering, afraid. Indeed, when we tuck our tail under like a dog we feel the floor of the pelvis narrow and tighten. Our hips clench, and breathing becomes restricted. "Wag your tail" and everything changes—the floor of the pelvis opens, the position of the pelvis shifts, and breathing opens and happens freely on its own. (This is only safe to do if the rib cage wheel is rolling forward too.)

The floor of the pelvis is a collection of hammocks strung in a crisscross pattern spanning various points of attachment on the pelvis. You can imagine what happens when these muscle fibers are continuously squeezed and tightened in an unbalanced way, pulling and misaligning their natural shape. This is not unlike setting a table with a beautiful tablecloth and fine china and crystal, then giving a tug to one corner of the tablecloth, causing all the table settings to go askew.

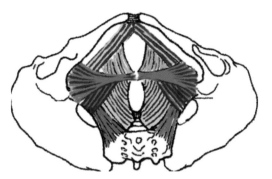

The pattern of muscles in the pelvic floor resembles an arrangement of hammocks.

Long-standing tension in pelvic floor muscles appears to play a role in some cases of pelvic floor myalgia, prostatitis, interstitial cystitis, and incontinence.[1] It appears there may well be a connection between these conditions and the position of the pelvis. Far-fetched? One example, among countless others, of how unquestioned assumptions about posture serve as blinders we wear in our approach to many common conditions is the fact that a tucked pelvis is accepted as being normal, even ideal. Pelvic pain, a surprisingly common condition in men, is often misdiagnosed as prostatitis, although closer examination reveals chronic tightness in pelvic floor muscles in the greatest majority of cases. While this has been tied by some health professionals to a human instinct to protect the genitals, the problem appears to be nonexistent in people who have a naturally anteverted pelvis, where pelvic floor muscles are more naturally relaxed. (See the exercise that follows.) If psychological factors are involved it seems more likely this results from entrenched excitation of the fear reflex, causing chronic tucking and tightening of the pelvic floor and iliopsoas (fear reflex) muscles. It would be hard to know which came first, the trauma that embedded fear in the musculature or the misalignment that generated the chronic tightening that also triggers low-level engagement of the fear reflex.

Of course it is never so simple and straightforward as this would suggest, yet skeletal alignment offers a likely explanation for why some people, over the long run, have found relief from these symptoms by learning to repeatedly anchor the pelvis in an anteverted position in everything they do. The position of the pelvis affects the position of vital organs, their various tubes and valves, pelvic muscles, including those of the pelvic floor, and the placement of undue pressure on nerve fibers within the pelvic region.

This would also explain why novelist Tim Parks, who found relief from pelvic floor pain by taking up the practice of meditation, went on to write *Teach Us to Sit Still,* a book that details Parks's journey in learning how to release deep tensions within his body.[2] Not only does meditation help train the mind to release mental tensions, but the correct sitting position for meditation puts the pelvis in the ante-verted position. As Parks wrote to me in a recent correspondence, "it is blindingly obvious that posture is important," even though this fact is largely overlooked by the medical profession in addressing these painful symptoms.[3] Were research to be conducted related to pelvic pain syndrome and its relationship to the position of the pelvis, it would not be surprising to discover that almost everyone presenting with these symptoms also presented with a chronically tucked pelvis.

TRY IT ON!

Ringing the Pelvic Bell

- It is helpful to do this standing sideways in front of a full-length mirror. Stand with your heels 6 inches apart and your toes 8 inches apart.
- Move your thighs forward, in front of you, then move them back behind you. Repeat this a few times, noticing how this causes your pelvis to swing back and forth like a bell swinging in a church tower.

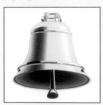

Picture your pelvis as a bell such as this.

- Notice that when the pubic bone moves forward and up the sitz bones slide forward and closer to each other. When the pubic bone moves down and slides out behind you the sitz bones move back and widen. *Caution:* Do not lift the sitz bones up behind you as this will cause unnecessary tension in the lower back and hips. Let them simply slide out straight behind you. Notice how the tailbone also moves along with the sitz bones and pubis.

- Repeat this movement slowly, paying close attention to any sensations you observe. These may include tightening and releasing of muscles in the front and back of the thighs, the hips joints, the buttocks, and the belly. Notice the sensations in the floor of the pelvis—how it tightens and narrows when the pubic bone rises up in front then opens and relaxes as the pubic bone moves down again.

- Do you notice how the position of your legs shifts, with your legs coming directly underneath you when your pubic bone aims behind your heels? If you feel unsteady and wobbly, relax your belly and lean your upper body forward. Your leg muscles are not accustomed to working in this way and will need time and practice to readjust to supporting you in this position. Hold on to a wall or the back of a chair if you feel unstable. Do *not* do this exercise if doing so causes you any pain.

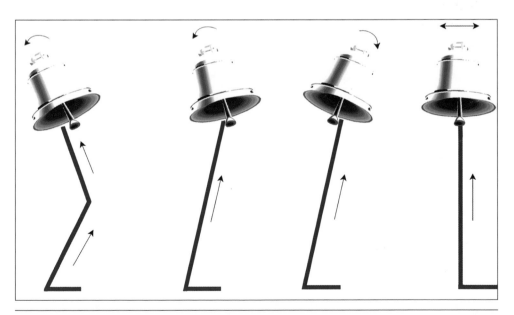

As you move through this exercise, notice how the position of your pelvis changes in the same way that these bells tilt forward and back.

TRY IT ON!

Ringing the Rib Cage Bell

- Sit with your feet flat on the floor and anchor your pelvis.
- Picture your rib cage as a large bell and begin to slowly ring the bell back and forth. This exploration greatly resembles the movements you explored in envisioning the rib cage as a turning wheel. Again, be sure that the pelvis does not move.

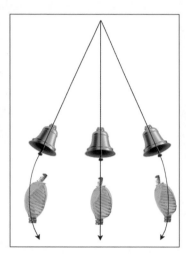

Note the marked shift in the position of the bells as your rib cage rotates to the front and back.

- Pay close attention to the shifting length in the lines along the front and then the back of your body (between the blue dots in the image below). As the bottom rim of the bell swings behind you the line in the front shortens and your back rounds; as the bottom rim of the bell swings to the front the back arches and the chest pushes out. *Caution:* Do not do this if you feel any pain!

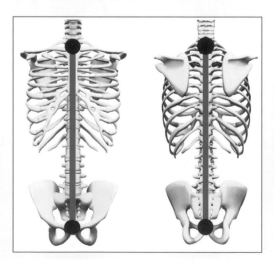

Imagine these lines on the front and back of your body and visualize how they lengthen and shorten as you move your rib cage.

- Can you feel your spine compress on whichever side the line is shortening? Can you find that middle place, where the line is the same length in the front and the back? Keep relaxing the belly. Are you able to tell that the spine is optimally extended when the line in the front and the line in the back are the same length?
- You may have to remind the superficial belly to relax to allow the pelvis and the rib cage to move independently of each other.

"A person who has been holding his chest high . . . feels when first told to disregard his chest in accordance with better mechanical adjustment, that he is losing some of his moral force by so doing. . . . Effective responses to new sensations and better coordinated action will bring about new habits, or new patterns of posture, which in time will feel comfortable."[4]

THE BELL ON TOP

The image of a bell works well for exploring the basic up-and-down (nodding *yes*) movement of the atlanto-occipital joint, where the head rests on top of the spine. When the bottom rim of the head bell swings forward the chin comes up; when the bell swings back the chin drops and the base of the skull rises behind. Notice too that the front of the throat moves toward the back of the neck.

Another way to experience the natural placement of the head is to imagine the

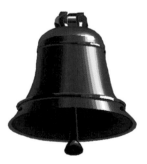

While you picture the up-and-down movement of the chin, visualize the head as this bell, with one edge representing the chin and the opposite edge representing the base of the skull.

top of the head being partially filled with sand. When you lift your chin the sand pours into the back of the head, and the weight of the sand bears down onto the spine.

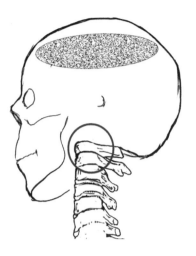

Imagining the top of the skull filled with a bowl of shifting sand helps to locate the point of balance where the muscles of the neck are relaxed.

TRY IT ON!

The Shifting Sands

- Slowly drop your chin toward your chest, just far enough to feel the imagined sand shift toward the front of the head. Stop just before the front of the throat begins to tighten. You are looking for the middle place where the sand is balanced between front and back and the muscles of the neck are optimally relaxed.

- Keep shifting the sand back and forth very slowly until this place becomes clear. In this position the cervical spine is fully elongated through the neck. It may actually feel like the sand is more toward the front when the neck muscles are most relaxed, especially if your habit is to have your chin lifted a bit. This may feel odd, because it is different from the position to which most of us are accustomed.

- It helps to picture the cluster of short muscles at the base of your skull at their full length, without being stretched out. The more you know about how the mechanism of your body works—and feels—the more you will be in the driver's seat of guiding your body to where it belongs. Relaxing your belly will help relax the neck.

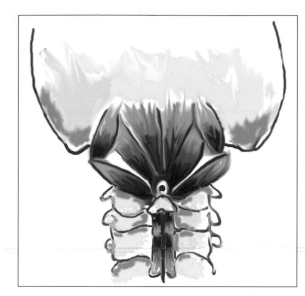

These small muscles attach at the topmost vertebrae and the occiput. They shorten as the chin rises and lengthen as the chin drops.

The more you explore these simple movements and tune in to the sensations associated with each one the more you will gain a deeper understanding of how your body works when it is most aligned, most relaxed, and most innately and solidly anchored. With this level of self-knowledge you will have the tools you need to protect yourself from injury and pain throughout your lifetime.

Knowing how to "sweep" the neck helps you put your head on straight. The key to this is to maintain the relationship of the rib cage to the pelvis so that the chest does not begin to lift as you roll the head wheel forward.

TRY IT ON!

Neck Sweep

The neck sweep is a subtle, gentle movement that is more of an imagined shift than it is an action that involves muscles.

- Anchor the pelvis.
- Turn on the power button.
- Begin by dropping your chin slightly. Think of the point at the front of your throat where an Adam's apple would be. Imagine this spot, without any muscle tension involved, sliding ever so gently toward the back of the throat and floating up the back of your neck.

- Imagine your ears like wheels, with the rim of the ears rolling up and forward as the cervical spine lengthens through the back of your neck. Remember this is

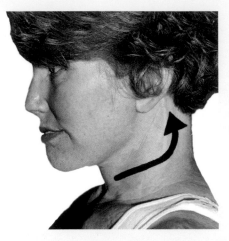

Gently rolling the head wheel forward in the neck sweep

feather soft and is guided more by thought than by muscle action.
- If you feel that your eyes are cast downward as a result of this, open your eyes wider in order to look up rather than lifting your chin. This will feel strange at first, because you will be using your eye muscles differently; but before long this will begin to feel more natural. Lifting the chin causes the eyelids to close slightly. Dropping your chin slightly means you will be looking out at the world with your eyes wide open!
- Exhale and relax.

SHOULDERING WEIGHT WITH EASE

The shoulders, like the arms and hands, legs and feet, are part of the appendicular skeleton, which consists of appendages to the main body. The pelvis, sacrum, spine, rib cage, and skull all make up the axial, or primary, skeleton. This can be misleading, because the shoulder girdle plays an essential role in tying the aligned skeleton together.

The shoulder girdle is comprised of three pairs of bones—the shoulder blades (*scapulae*), collarbones (*clavicles*), and upper arm bones (*humerus*). The actions of these three bones work together in an ingenious way that gives the shoulder remarkable stability while also offering the widest range of motion of any joint in the body.

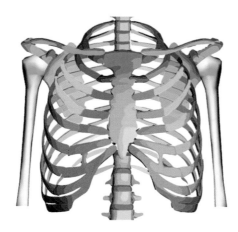

The bones that form
the shoulder girdle

The clavicle works somewhat like a yoke, drawing its greatest strength not from the muscles around it but from an efficient, load-distributing biotensegrity mechanism. If the shoulder bones slip off their perch on top of the rib cage the whole system becomes unstable, forcing the load onto the muscles.

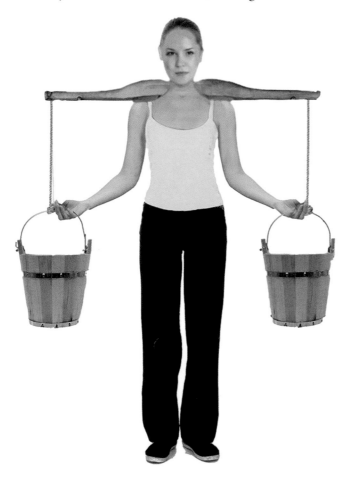

The clavicles stabilize
the shoulder girdle and
distribute weight in the
same way this yoke
provides stability so this
woman can more easily
carry her burden.

As seen in the photos below, misalignment of the shoulder girdle is the most common reason many people experience shoulder pain and chronic shoulder tension. Nevertheless the axial skeleton has to be set up and aligned before the shoulders can snap into place, which is why discussion of the shoulders has been saved until last.

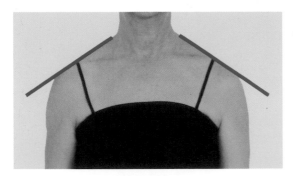

Pulling the shoulders down distorts the shoulder girdle, restricts mobility, and puts a drag on the *trapezius* and *levator scapulae* muscles.

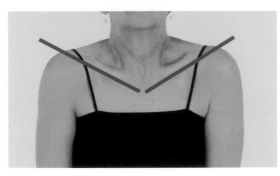

Lifting the shoulders or rolling them forward breaks the angle of the collarbones and tightens the muscles.

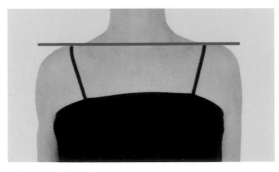

When the collarbone is placed in its solid yoke-like position muscles are elastic, and shoulders are level and able to enjoy the full range of motion.

Shoulders with overdeveloped muscles dramatically restrict range of motion. While muscle strength makes it possible to lift heavy objects in prescribed ways, the movement of the shoulder blades is restricted by bulky muscles that limit the shoulder's ability to move with natural flexibility. Excessive muscle tension in and around the shoulder girdle plays a big part in restricting the natural range of motion of the shoulder as well as contributing to chronic shoulder tension.

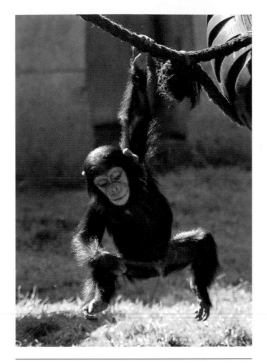

This photo of a young chimpanzee reveals a shoulder mechanism not unlike that of humans. This is not surprising, because chimpanzees and humans share more than 98 percent identical DNA, and chimpanzees and bonobos appear to be our closest relatives in the animal kingdom.[5]

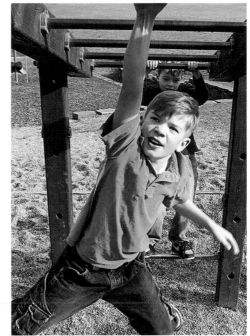

This may explain why human children enjoy swinging on monkey bars at the playground. This boy is swinging hand over hand (from branch to branch). This action is called brachiating and is characteristic of apes. Monkeys do not brachiate, actually, but jump and run along branches, meaning that monkey bars might be more accurately called "ape bars."

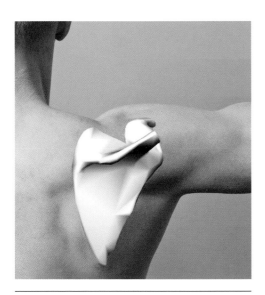

This depiction shows how bulky muscles could bind the free movement of the shoulder.

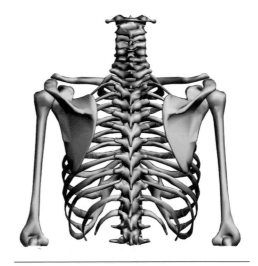

The shoulder blades, seen here from the back, rest on the back of the rib cage and move in sync with the clavicle and top of the arm bone.

PAT YOURSELF ON THE BACK

The shoulder blades can be pictured as two hands on your back. With this image in mind the bottom of each scapula becomes the heel of the hand. Bend one arm with your hand by your shoulder and the elbow by your waist. Move the elbow slowly through the air. Notice when the elbow goes out behind you that your shoulder rolls forward. Can you sense how the "heel of the hand" lifts away from the rib cage? Moving your elbow forward of the center reconnects the bottom of the shoulder blade with your rib cage and secures your shoulder in place. Do not lift your chest as you do this. Teach yourself how to isolate the movement of the shoulders from the rib cage so that you're not displacing the rib cage and the spine to which it is attached every time you reach for something.

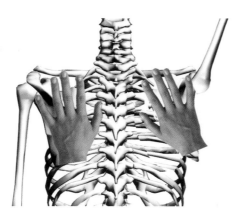

Visualize the shoulder blades as two hands on your back as shown here.

As you continue to move your elbow in wider circles you'll begin to understand more how the shoulder mechanism works and how you can isolate shoulder movements from the rib cage. You'll soon realize that keeping the core engaged is the key. Good flexibility in the shoulder makes it possible for you to reach a book from a high shelf, to swing a tennis racket or baseball bat, or to swim using different strokes, but it's core strength that helps to keep the shoulder in check so that it is stable and protected in such movements.

TRY IT ON!

Fasten the Shoulders

- Anchor the pelvis.
- Turn on the power button.
- Now roll one shoulder at a time up, around, and back (but not down) so that

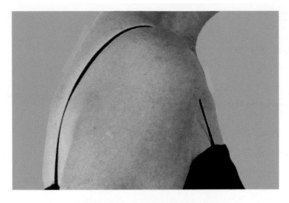

Shoulder dropped
forward of rib cage

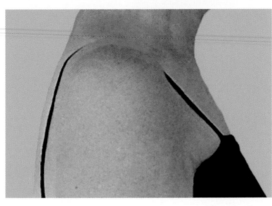

Aligned shoulder resting
on top of rib cage

the shoulder comes to rest directly on top of the rib cage, and the elbow is at
the back of the waist.

- At first this should be done one shoulder at a time. Over time, as you become
better able to keep the rib cage stationary (power button turned on) so that the
chest will not lift even the smallest amount, you can begin to practice moving
both shoulders on to the top of the rib cage at the same time.

It helps to know that you can rotate the palm of your hand without moving
the upper arm or shoulder as the action takes place below the elbow. This can feel
strange at first if you are in the habit of moving your hand by moving your shoulder. You can practice moving your arms around and doing certain activities with
your shoulder blades remaining in place on your back. Knowing how to keep the
shoulders stabilized can help you learn to release chronic shoulder strain and tension. Following are a few exercises that can help you with this.

TRY IT ON!

Exercises to Save the Shoulders

These simple exercises accomplish a lot, from relieving chronic tension in the shoulders to repairing rotator cuff injuries that usually require surgery. The key here is fastening the shoulders and training muscles to keep the shoulder girdle stabilized.

- Stand close to a wall and place your elbows on the wall at shoulder level, with your forearms and hands extending straight up from the elbows.

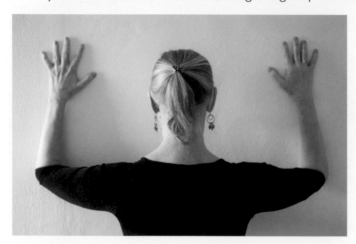

This is the correct position for beginning this exercise.

- Hold on to the wall with your hands as you begin to draw your elbows toward each other. You will feel some action around the shoulder blades as they secure into place.

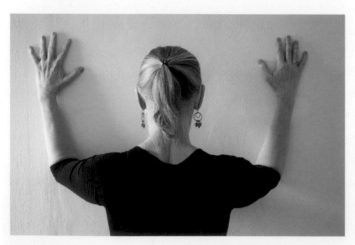

This is the position you will be in when you have completed the movement. Note that the shoulder blades have moved closer together.

This simple movement often brings almost instant relief from a host of shoulder complaints.

- Another way to do this is to hold a dowel or broomstick behind your head at the base of the skull (occiput).

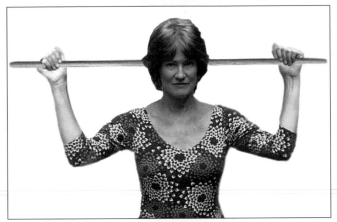

Note the position of the dowel or broomstick at the base of the skull, not behind the neck.

- Holding on to the stick, draw your elbows toward each other, as if trying to touch them together in front of you.
- You can simultaneously use the stick to draw the occiput upward, inviting length into the back of the neck.
- Do all of these exercises often, and your shoulders will thank you.

Here's one final trick to help train the shoulders to stay in place.

- Begin by rolling your shoulders, one at a time, up, around, and back so that your shoulder blades fasten onto the back of the rib cage (as we learned in the fasten the shoulder exercise).
- Turn your palms up and place the back (bony part) of your elbows at the front of your waist.

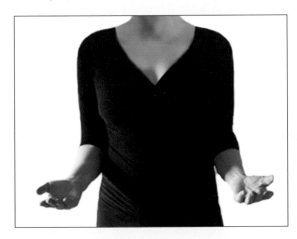

Note that the elbows are held close to the body.

- If you are able to just sit for a while, such as at a movie or concert, let the backs of your hands rest on your thighs.

As your muscles acclimate to this way of being, tight muscles will loosen and overlengthened muscles will firm up. You can turn your palms down by keeping your elbows attached to your waist and rotating the lower arms below the elbows. If you are able to place a computer keyboard on a low tray or position a laptop so that your hands can remain here, this is an ideal position for typing—while sitting on an anchored pelvis, of course.

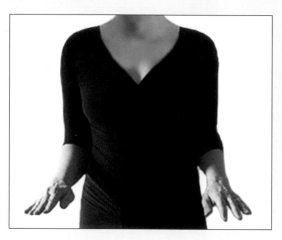

This is the ideal position for typing while maintaining the shoulders in a relaxed position.

PULLING YOUR OWN STRINGS

Imagining yourself to be a puppet, and simultaneously the puppeteer, provides you with many useful tools. A tense dog puppet is pulled up by taut strings that represent the tension required to hold a misaligned body upright. If that tension is loosened, misaligned bones are unable to provide structural support, the strings go slack, and the body collapses into a sad dog stance. Attaching imaginary strings at strategic places on the back of the body draws the body back on to the axis, where the bones align and are able to support the upright body without unnecessary tension. In fact, there is almost a sense of the body hanging effortlessly from above at the same time that it is deeply planted into the earth through solid, aligned legs.

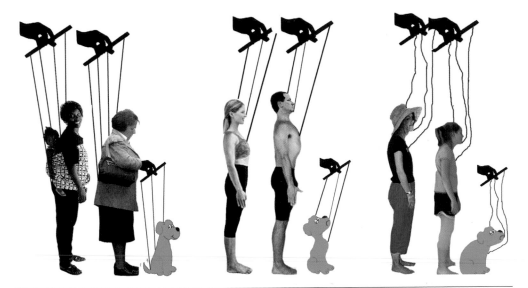

Note how the happy dog stance on the left is neither pulled forward with unnecessary tension or collapsing, unsupported, as are the tense dog and sad dog stances.

When the body is aligned along the axis it is easy to imagine puppet strings attached, from the bottom up:

- on each sitz bone
- at the bottom of either side of the rib cage
- just under the back of each armpit
- inside the front of each armpit
- at the base of the skull

The puppeteer draws the entire body back to the center of the axis, lengthening the back upward. This takes a bit of practice, but it is more than worthwhile. As you work with this image you will come to feel the puppet strings drawing you back to center as well as engaging the core and elongating the spine.

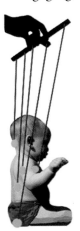

The green dots identify the contact points of the imaginary puppet strings maintaining an aligned body.

AN EXPLODING CRISIS IN CHILDREN'S HEALTH

NOWHERE IS THERE more urgency for research that examines the details of the human body's natural design than as it relates to the mushrooming health crisis among children today. We have to ask why, when so many children in the "advanced" world are struggling with a long list of physical complaints and health issues, many other children in the world are able to carry heavy loads on their heads with ease, seemingly without developing either chronic pain problems or neurodevelopmental disorders.

Certainly no suggestion is being made here that children should all start carrying heavy things on their heads, but we miss the boat by ignoring clues related to this that may well have a bearing on some of the health problems facing so many children today. All children are, after all, the exact same species.

We tend to think of children in such places as Africa and India as far less healthy and privileged than children in our country, who enjoy many modern benefits. Research, were it to be conducted on this subject, would probably reveal that there are far fewer cases of developmental disabilities and neurological disorders among those children who routinely participate in village and family life by doing physical tasks, such as carrying water on their heads, than are seen in the United States today. While many children in the undeveloped world are facing terrible conditions—poverty, hunger, exploitation, abuse, and illness due to poor sanitary conditions and communicable diseases, it may still be a mistake to assume that children who carry water on their heads or siblings on their backs, as many of them have done for generations, are being exploited or suffering. In fact, it may

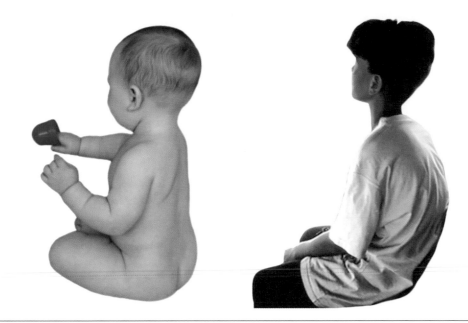

Virtually all babies start with aligned spines, yet as seen here that alignment can quickly be lost.

turn out that these children have at least some advantages that children do not have when they live in modern societies that have lost their way. Are we fooling ourselves in touting our many advancements while not recognizing that we have unwittingly failed our children by leaving so many of them "disembodied" and physically disempowered?

The children pictured on the following page are but a sampling of children elsewhere in the world who easily carry heavy loads of water on their heads. Many of these children will grow up to continue to carry water and other heavy items on their heads, some for decades to come, without developing spinal problems. American children have no need to carry heavy loads on their heads, but they do need to live in bodies that share the same skeletal alignment that makes this possible.

Americans have seen the rate of autism rise from one in ten thousand children only forty years ago, to one in eighty-eight children in the year 2012. The sharpest climb has been in the past decade. While changing criteria for making diagnoses may have played a part in this jump, there is an undeniable epidemic that is growing rapidly, with no end in sight. Sometimes called neurodevelopmental disorders, sensory processing disorders, or sensory integration dysfunction, they reveal themselves in conditions commonly known as the autism spectrum disorders and range from severe autism to high-functioning autism, or Asperger's syndrome. Some of

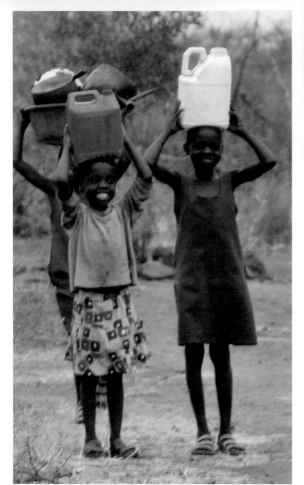
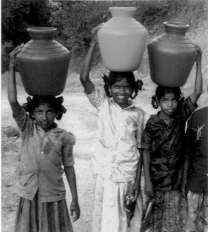
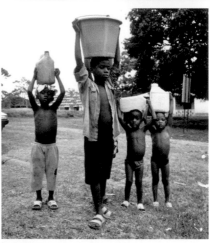
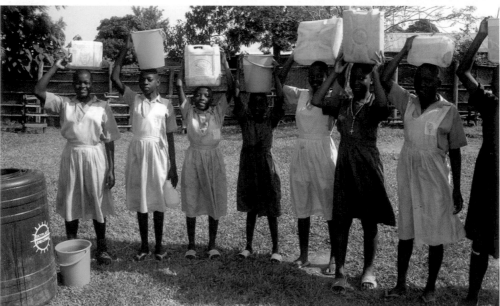

The weight of the load is comfortably distributed through aligned spines that are supported atop an anteverted pelvis and legs that serve as vertical pillars of support.

these symptoms overlap with other disorders that have also skyrocketed in number, including ADHD (attention deficit hyperactivity disorder), bipolar disorder, Tourette's syndrome, OCD (obsessive compulsive disorder), childhood schizophrenia, and depression. It is now being suggested these may all be different manifestations of the same underlying neurodevelopmental condition. Although ADHD was first described as long ago as the mid-1800s, the incidence of this condition remained very rare, with mention of isolated cases popping up in medical literature every decade or so. Today one in ten children has some form of ADHD, with the numbers rising between 3 percent and 5 percent per year.[1]

The numbers are staggering. While changes in diagnostic procedures may account for some of the cases, they don't begin to explain the overwhelming epidemic that has turned family and classroom life upside down. Many children who are considered healthy by today's lowered standards still struggle with delayed physical development, low muscle tone, sleep disorders, anxiety, excessive weight, vision dysfunction, recurring stress injuries, poor flexibility, chronic fatigue, and unexplained pain. The picture this paints is alarming, to say the least.

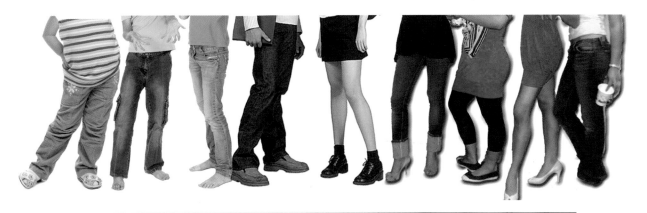

Young people today have developed a wide range of postural habits and are beset with poor alignment.

COMMAND CENTRAL RUN AMOK

Most of the problems facing children share some type of disruption of what would be normal functioning of the nervous system. We tend to think of the nervous system as primarily the brain, which acts as the processing center that interprets and responds to neural impulses. Just as important, however, may be the other half of the central nervous system, the spinal cord. This "forgotten brain" is the primary neural pathway for the transmission of messages through countless nerve fibers that relay instructions from the brain by way of motor neurons and back to the brain by way of sensory neurons. Nobel laureate and neurobiologist Roger Sperry suggested that the spinal cord is the engine that drives the brain.[2] According to Sperry, "90% of stimulation and nutrition to the brain is generated by the movement of the spine."

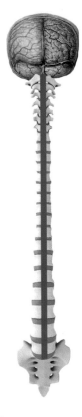

The brain and the spinal cord form the central nervous system.

The brain has also been compared to the control tower at a busy international airport, processing and integrating information as it comes in for a landing and sending out light-speed instructions for coordinating takeoffs. Imagine how little the brain would have to do if there were no planes taking off or landing, or how dysfunctional the brain might become if all the planes' messages were scrambled—or worse yet, actually crashing.

It appears that something like this is taking place with neurodevelopmental disorders and unintegrated primitive reflexes. While there may be any number of underlying causes for these conditions—genetics, chemicals in the environment, toxins in immunizations, additives in food, prenatal factors, birth trauma, allergies, gluten sensitivity, electromagnetic radiation—years of study have not identified any one of these as a certain cause.

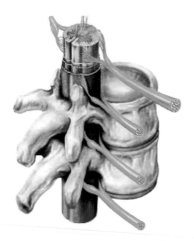

The spine protects the spinal cord, from which nerve fibers extend throughout the body sending and receiving electrical impulses.

One possible cause stands out for the fact that it has been thoroughly overlooked: disruption of the human body's naturally unfolding process of physical development in the earliest months or years of life. We may have failed to understand the details of a universal process taking place in children and the devastating effects that can result from disruption of this process. Of course there is no hard evidence yet that this is so, but there is a lot of compelling information, much of it presented here, that demands that this be more closely examined.

STAYING CONNECTED

To better understand this, let's take a look at what occurs from the time a baby is born. It has been suggested that human infants, being the most helpless of all mammals for the longest period of time, are born at nine-months gestation so that the growing head can still fit through the birth canal. Mothers throughout the world, by wearing their babies in slings and wrapping them onto their bodies, have traditionally created an external "kangaroo pouch" that, in many cultures, appears to extend the gestational period into a beyond-the-womb phase. This practice, which has most likely been maintained for thousands of years, has kept babies in perpetual physical contact with their mothers. If they are put down alone it is not for long. They sleep alongside their mothers and often other members of the family as well. These mothers understand, as if by instinct, an abiding human connection with the natural world and the physical nurturing that is shared among all mother and baby mammals.

Jean Liedloff, who lived among Stone Age Indians in South America over a period of five years, believed that a sustained "in-arms" experience was necessary for healthy physical and emotional development in children.[3] Her pioneering work laid the foundation for the rise of attachment parenting, a movement that has grown in popularity among some parents in recent years. Liedloff wrote that the Yequana children she observed in the Venezuelan jungle were calm and cheerfully obedient, they were undemanding and never whined, and they would play easily together without conflict, all while exhibiting empathy and compassion at a young age. It stands to reason that mental and emotional health is related to physical health in many ways, and while Liedloff's findings are more suggestive than conclusive, this line of thinking allows us to draw a further possible connection between indigenous child-rearing practices and conformance with a natural physical design.

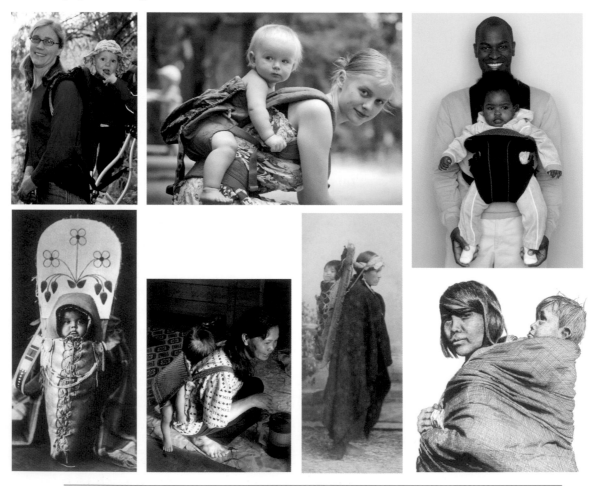

Photographs from around the world reveal how mothers in many cultures employed, and in some cases both parents continue to employ, practices that preserved the integrity of the baby's spine, even if they were unaware that this is what they were doing.

In wearing a baby in a sling, the adult's own position at any given time placed the baby directly onto its own aligned pelvis, and the baby bending forward simply shifted the weight to the front of the baby's own body in a "belly-to-earth" experience. Rarely, if ever, was the baby's weight put onto the back of the pelvis, as is so commonly done today. Joined with the parent in this way, if curious about what was going on and wanting to participate in looking around more actively, the baby would have to enlist ground reaction force by pushing off in a way that anchored the pelvis downward and elongated the spine. This would occur simultaneously, a bit like two elevators in one shaft, one going down, the other going up. This action triggered the internal core that the baby would need for all future milestones—sitting, crawling, standing, and walking.

BACK TO FRONT

Until recently infants in modern Western society, although seldom worn by their mothers, spent much of their earliest months lying on their stomachs, enabling them to engage downward in order to develop this essential core from which movement is initiated. Over the past two decades this practice has changed dramatically.

Today many babies in our culture spend almost all of their time, waking and sleeping, either lying on their backs or in a semireclining position. Life, for the youngest of babies, is often lived in a succession of carriers—car seats, strollers, bouncy seats, swings, and other such devices that place their weight on the back of the pelvis.

Babies enter the world with a complex nervous system in place, with all the necessary working parts ready to go but not yet test-driven. Like laying tracks for the coming railroad, it appears that neural pathways are developed through a step-by-step process that systematically fires up synapses between neurons that turns on this fledgling nervous system by way of a baby's earliest movements. Babies drive this sequential flow through exercising the body, updating information, and processing events that apparently build one upon the other. These developmental stages don't just magically happen. The baby must do the work of developing a dynamic physical self. This is the work of all species' babies, to fulfill a deep, biologically driven impulse to develop and thrive. A big part of a human baby doing this job is building a powerful core of stability that supports an elongated spine and helps control traffic flowing freely through the information superhighway, or spinal cord.

TRY IT ON!

Be a Baby Again

- Take a moment to lie down on your stomach on a bed or the floor. (If that's not possible right now, *imagine* you are doing this as you read through the exercise, and then go through it again later when you can lie down.)
- Place one or two standard-size bed pillows, laid lengthwise, under your torso. Your head should be off the pillow and turned to the side. Draw your chin down slightly to lengthen the back of your neck.
- Bend your hips and knees into a modified frog legs position, mimicking the way a baby would lie on his belly. This will protect your back from arching.
- Pretend that you are brand new to the world and have almost no muscle tone. You are powerless to lift your very heavy head up off the surface that is under you.
- Ask yourself—what has to happen in order for me to be able to lift this heavy head? What do I have to do to make this happen?
- It doesn't take long to realize that you have to engage with the ground by pushing down in order to trigger a rising response in your body that comes from engaging ground reaction force (GRF). Engage all of your body, not just your arms or legs, with the surface on which you are lying.

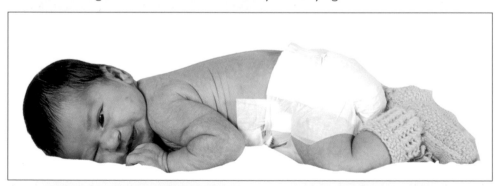

Like this baby, you must begin to push against the ground to enable your body to rise up.

- Continue to initiate this movement, ever so slightly, in tiny micromovements.
- Notice where you are feeling the response in your body. Are you feeling it in your arms and legs? Do you feel it along your back and spine? Do you sense your spine lengthening and opening? Do you feel a firming of the core muscles of the abdomen as you bear down? This is what babies are experiencing too, and one can only imagine what they are thinking about it all!

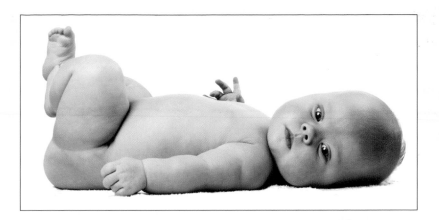

Lying on the back, a newborn is unable to engage ground reaction force to build the essential core needed to lift the head.

- Now turn over onto your back.
- How successfully can you engage with the ground beneath you in this position? Can you sense how your movements are pretty much restricted to just moving your arms and legs through space, without much sense of turning on a mysterious connection throughout your body? Do you think you could develop much core strength lying in this position? Do you think that if you were in this position, in a car seat or baby swing for most of every day, that, over time, it would be somewhat physically disempowering?

Healthy babies know what to do. Instinct guides them through a specific series of milestones, both large and small, driven by an impulse to work relentlessly to fulfill their bodies' promise. Babies follow a more or less prescribed sequence of exercises that appear to turn on the nervous system, strengthen muscles, and generate a specific pattern of mechanical movement shared by all natural humans. While the actions of a baby may appear, at first glance, to be random and unfocused, they are defined by a drive toward acquiring the strength, coordination, and balance needed to succeed in becoming upright.

Only a few decades ago most babies spent quite a bit of time in a belly-to-earth position. Today, with few opportunities to become familiar with this position, some babies become upset when put on their tummies. They cry in what appears to be frustration at not having the core stability needed to hold up their heads, causing them to feel uncomfortable in this position.

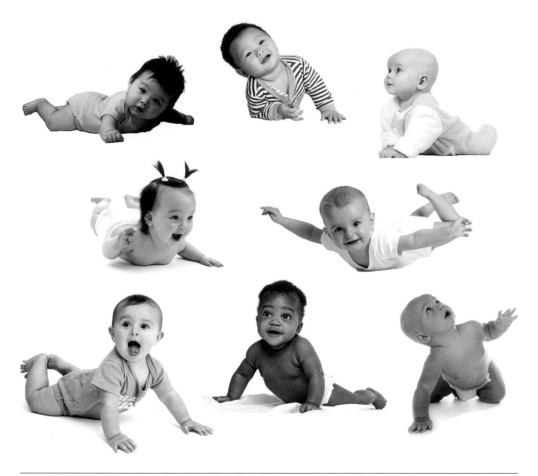

Key to the process of learning to sit up, crawl, stand, and walk is deep engagement at the core, intended to stabilize an upright spine for a whole lifetime. This occurs when the little body pushes down on the crib mattress or blanket on the floor, either of which serves to represent the earth, in an equal exchange between direct action (baby pushing down) and GRF (response in the body).

For this reason practices such as rolling up a towel under the baby's chest or using a specially manufactured "tummy time mat" to prop up the baby have recently come into use. Doing this should be avoided under all circumstances. A baby's job at this stage is to be actively working to develop the core, so essential to sensory and motor development. While it is not recommended that babies be left to cry or be miserable, some frustration, as evidenced in the hard work expended by the babies of other species, appears to be part of a mechanism for driving a baby's development toward the next milestone. Engaged belly-to-earth activity is required to build a robust and enlivened body and brain.

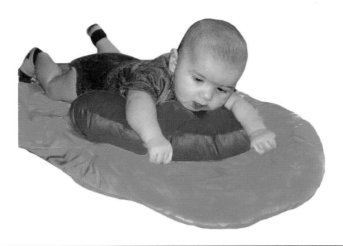

Propping a baby up this way interferes with the important stage of developing the core and may spell trouble later. The more we interfere with the natural, baby-led process that is driven by the instincts of our species, the more we run into problems.

If a baby has not had an opportunity to become accustomed to a stomach position, the best thing to do is to lie down on your stomach facing the baby. Babies are so eager to interact with us this often keeps them happily engaged in this position, at least for a few minutes. You can build up the time by doing this in short spurts until your baby is actively enjoying the workout routine that a growing and developing body needs. In some instances more remedial measures may be necessary.

The problem is not just riding in a car seat or sleeping in a slumped position from time to time. Problems develop when supine or semisupine activities are frequently strung together to constitute a large part of a baby's daily life. These are the activities that kill the core. Eliminating car seats is obviously not an option. With a new understanding of postural rules, car seat manufacturers could begin to make it a priority to design these devices to support a baby's spine, awake or asleep. They need not worry about sales; millions of conscientious parents will snatch them up.

At any given moment we, as parents, are either supporting our baby's naturally unfolding development or we are preventing it. Having little information available about this fact has caused the unwitting creation of serious health problems for many children.

In an effort to lower the incidence of SIDS (sudden infant death syndrome) the American Academy of Pediatrics launched the 1992 "Back to Sleep" campaign

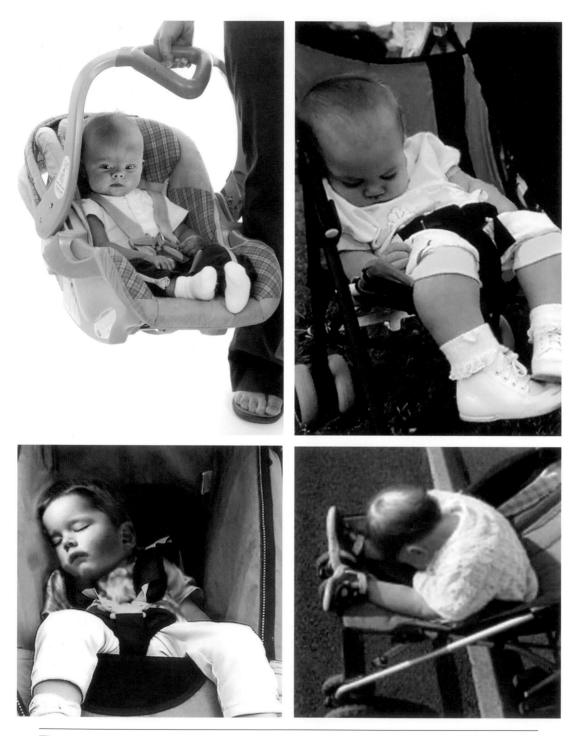

The average stroller, car seat, or carrier does not support a baby's spine and simultaneously places far too much pressure on the back of the pelvis and deprives the baby of the opportunity to develop core strength.

that recommended that all babies be put on their backs to sleep at all times.[4] This has planted a seed in parents' minds that, if babies should be sleeping on their backs, maybe it is better, generally, for them to be in this position. Coupled with the growing dependence on devices such as car seats, strollers, and swings, all of which put babies in a semireclining position with their tailbones tucked under, this more modern approach has given way to a new "on the back" existence for many babies today.

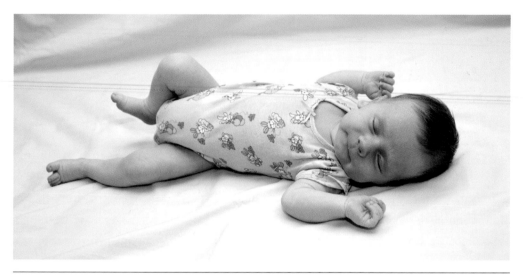

In an attempt to reduce the occurrence of SIDS, many parents have opted to position their infants on the back while sleeping and awake.

Often baby seats, swings, and floor mats have colorful objects dangling overhead that are used to entertain babies, with the idea of giving a baby's somewhat "empty" mind a head start in developing cognitive skills and a capacity for higher learning. Meanwhile, the importance of babies' physical development has been misunderstood, leaving many babies with bodies that have skipped the essential work of building the essential core of well-being that builds a nervous system capable of integrating and processing what may otherwise be experienced as a bombardment of external stimulation. Can it be that the very measures we are taking to enhance our children's lives are actually having the opposite effect? Are we also sending babies a message that what is "out there" is more important than what is "in here?"

The "Back to Sleep" campaign and the overreliance on sitting devices has led to a large jump in the number of babies with positional *plagiocephaly,* or flat-head syndrome.[5] Rarely seen a few generations ago, it is not uncommon today for the back of a baby's head to become flattened during the first six months. This new phenomenon is a direct result of babies spending an excessive amount of time lying on their backs or reclining in sitting devices. Some babies wear orthotic helmets around the clock to reshape their heads back to normal.

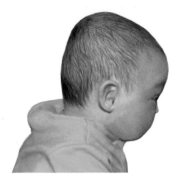

Too much time lying on the back actually causes the baby's head to become flattened.

Far more serious is the lack of core development in babies, as seen in the number of infants who display head lag when their arms are lifted from a supine position. Now seen as a sign of future developmental problems in some children, this is blamed on neck weakness, but the real culprit is a missing core. By the time babies are able to sit, crawl, stand, and walk upright those healthy babies who have spent much of the time on their stomachs will have almost all the core strength they will ever need.

Beyond six months of age, head lag is a clear symptom of insufficient core strength, development of which requires that the babies experience significant

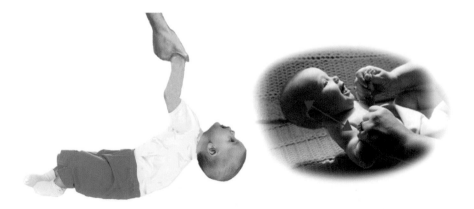

When a newborn is lifted by the hands from a lying to a sitting position it is normal for the head to flop back in a position commonly called *head lag*. By four months of age, most naturally developing babies have developed enough core strength to hold the head in line with the spine.

time on their stomachs. Remarkably, a recent study has revealed that 90 percent of all children diagnosed with autism at age three or four showed evidence of head lag at six months of age![6]

Supervised tummy time is now recommended by most pediatricians, in short bursts totaling thirty minutes a day, often to avoid developing a flat head. Unfortunately, the necessity of physical activity in the first several months is so essential to a child's normal physical development that thirty minutes appears to be far too little, and, in some cases, it comes too late.[7] While some children are able to catch up, others never do.

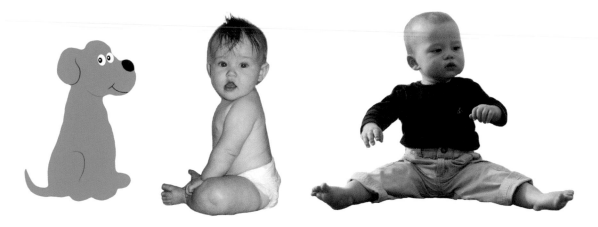

The human design for a deeply rooted, well-anchored pelvis is clearly evident in the babies pictured here. With such a solid foundation, the spine is able to stack up through the back in a perfect display of the dynamic interplay between aligned bones and elastic muscles—the happy dog stance.

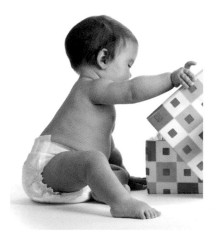

When a baby bends naturally, the whole pelvis tips forward, taking a long, straight spine with it.

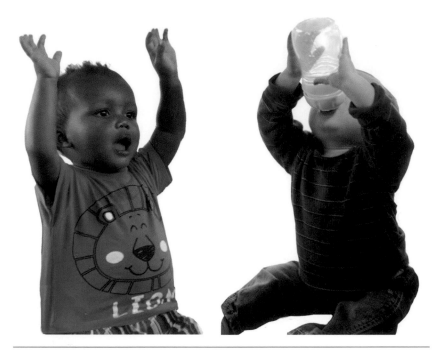

With an aligned pelvis solidly anchored, babies are able to raise their arms overhead, while keeping the spine elongated and intact.

CRAWLING, WALKING, AND SQUATTING

Many elements must come together for crawling to be mastered. Try as one might, a baby will not be able to crawl until adequate core strength has been developed to support the torso in a horizontal plane. Once the baby can master lifting up and balancing on all fours, the next big challenge becomes how to shift weight and balance with one arm or one leg lifted off the floor. If the pelvis and rib cage are placed in an unnatural relationship to each other, other muscles will have to adapt and start working in a dysfunctional way, disrupting the core.

Many babies are ingenious at developing personal styles of locomotion such as scooting backward or sliding across the floor on their bottoms, but sooner or later most babies do learn to coordinate the crisscross arm and leg pattern of bona-fide crawling.

By the time a well-developing baby has mastered sitting up, a deep core of stability that comes from an interplay of aligned bones and elastic postural muscles is the basis of internal support. What comes next—walking—adds the daring element of balance, which calls on the baby to align all the parts of the skeleton in

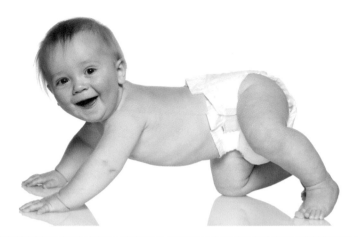

Success! This baby is well on the way to a full-fledged crawl.

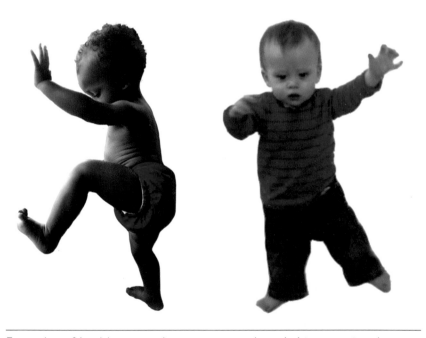

Examples of healthy, natural movement as these babies practice the balance necessary to take those first steps.

a precise relationship to the vertical axis in order to be able to balance a heavy "bowling ball" on top. This takes practice.

Squatting with heels on the floor and a long, open spine comes easily to babies and toddlers. If they remain aligned in the years ahead they will be able to squat with ease all the way into old age.

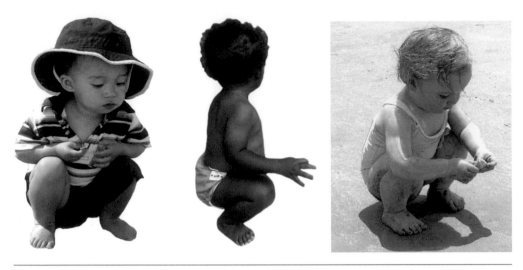

These very young children squat easily with flexible hips and aligned spines.

Often, years of misalignment result in a loss of the ability to comfortably squat for any length of time. Squatting in and of itself is not a prerequisite for hips that are flexible and free of compression. Rather, flexible hips are a prerequisite for squatting. While it is not necessary that everyone be able to squat or carry heavy loads on their heads. It is important to learn ways to inhabit the body in many different activities that encourage letting go of tensions that systematically bring newfound freedom of movement to compressed joints, thus returning us to the state enjoyed by babies and toddlers.

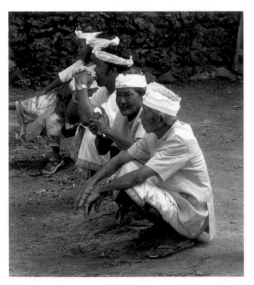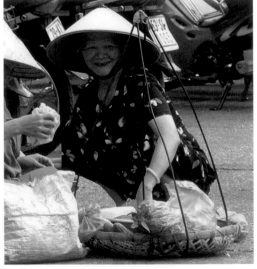

These adults exhibit the same ease and flexibility in squatting displayed by the very young.

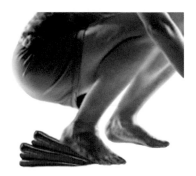

Folding a blanket or towel under the heels is a helpful way to encourage passive release of tightness in hips, knees, and ankles while dropping the weight of the pelvis onto the heels.

At some point, parents and others may begin to make note of cascading anomalies in a child's development. One such anomaly might be a failure to cross the midline, meaning a failure of the pelvis and rib cage to move independent of each other and disruption in the circuitry between the body and the brain. Atypical movement patterns reveal a lack of bilateral coordination that is a sign of weak core stability: the ankles are pronated, the knees rolled in (medially rotated), the pelvis tucked, the back rounded, the back of the head dropped back. None of these, by themselves, spell trouble, but many of them together could. Other signals might arise that are sometimes characteristic of a weak core unable to support a well-functioning nervous system—such as a child continuously seeking stimulation or just the opposite, withdrawing from an unbearable overload of stimulation that can't be integrated. A child might have difficulty mastering fine motor activities or show a deficiency in developing behavioral or social skills.

There are many exceptions, of course, but overall a healthy baby is one who inhabits a body that conforms to all the natural physical laws that support easeful mechanical movements and a thriving neural highway that travels through the spine.

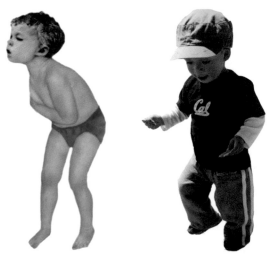

The child on the left is exhibiting unnatural movement patterns. The child on the right is exhibiting healthy, natural movement.

GROWING TREND TOWARD
UNHEALTHY SITTING

It is disheartening, to say the least, to see so many very young children lose pelvic support at the beginning of their lives. This very recent development among the youngest children appears to be caused by unnatural shortening of the rectus abdominis and psoas muscles and loss of essential toning and elasticity in the transversus abdominis. This is the outcome of a backward tilted pelvis, although only after adequate research has been conducted will the real culprit be named: too much time spent in the early months lying on the back and in a semireclining position to be able to build the essential core. It's likely that this trend plays a part in a whole menu of resulting problems that range from a delay in learning how to sit, crawl, stand, and walk, to full-blown developmental disorders that will plague some children for a lifetime.

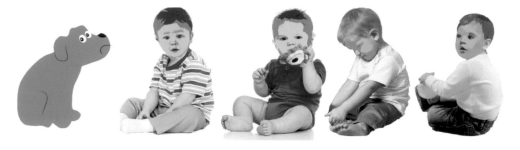

These children are already experiencing the lack of a core strong enough to support them in an aligned position and are in the slumped, sad dog stance.

Another unfortunate development is *W* sitting, common among children who have lost pelvis and core support. This position causes an extreme and unnatural rotation of the thighbone (femur) within the hip socket (*acetabulum*). This is a prescription for hip and knee surgery sometime down the road, a road that is getting shorter for the growing number of young adults who are having record numbers of surgeries to address what orthopedic surgeons routinely refer to as an underlying defect or dysplasia in the hip joint. This unnatural rotation of the femur also puts tremendous stress on the knees and contributes to pronation of the ankle and flat-footedness. These are serious problems that won't magically resolve themselves in the years ahead.

Not many generations ago, children sat on an anchored pelvis without having to be told what to do. The various systems of the body probably worked efficiently, including the circulatory system responsible for getting oxygenated blood to the brain, thus enhancing students' ability to focus and learn.

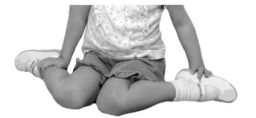
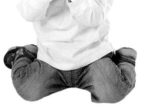
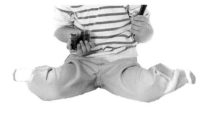

This position can give the false impression that the pelvis is anchored correctly, but someone trying to sit this way with a naturally rotated pelvis will find it extremely uncomfortable.

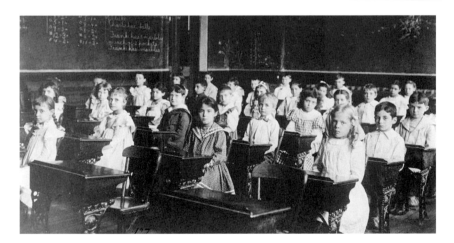

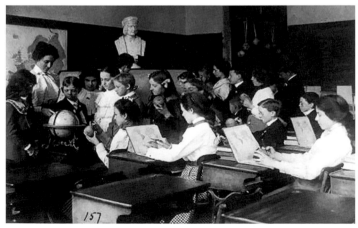
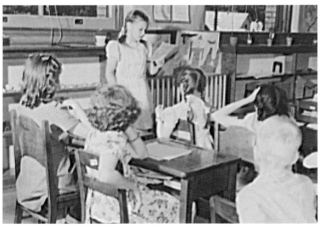

Although to our modern-day eyes these children may appear rigid and stiff, in actuality they are comfortably relaxed when supported by aligned bones.

Simply telling a child to "sit up straight" does little to solve the problem.

Typically, at the sound of these oft-repeated words, children lift up their chests, holding themselves up with tension in muscles that tire quickly. Within just moments they sink down into collapse again.

Only by learning how to anchor the pelvis and tether the rib cage into place with an engaged core can a child successfully sit up with comfort and ease. The good news is that children who have participated in pilot projects have demonstrated that they enjoy learning how their bodies are intended to work as much

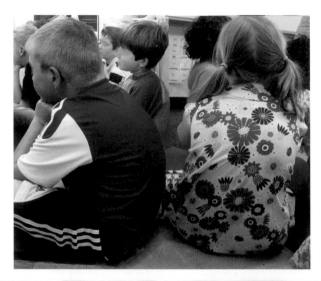

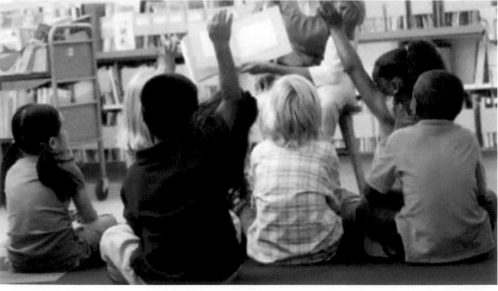

This slumped posture is common and cannot be resolved without engaging the core.

as they love learning how to sit comfortably, without effort and struggle.

Once lost, natural alignment can only be regained by a conscious, self-directed process by each individual making deliberate changes from the inside out. Sadly, because of chronic tucking under of the pelvis, it doesn't take long for many children to lose the support of aligned bones.

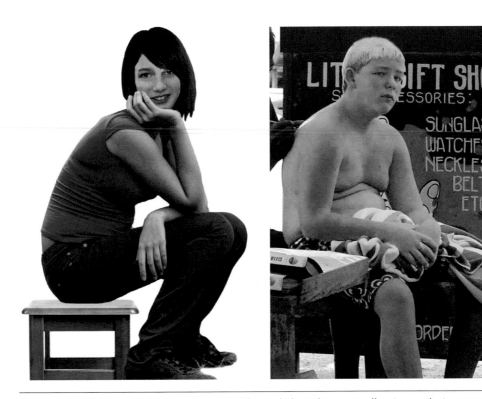

These two children have become so collapsed that they actually sit on their sacrum and tailbone (*coccyx*) rather than the front edge of the sitz bones. Their spines are severely deformed in this position, seriously distorting the spinal cord and putting pressure on nerve roots that pass through it. This puts the entire nervous system under assault. These children's bones are still growing, and unnatural weight distribution through their bones could well affect the way their bones grow.

This tucking of the tailbone is the root cause of the ever-growing epidemic of structural collapse that children are facing all over the world. Such collapsed posture causes their vital organs to be compressed to the point where functions relating to respiration, digestion, circulation, assimilation of nutrients, and elimination of waste are seriously affected. Most parents, teachers, and health professionals are unaware of the seriousness of this problem—and if they are aware of it, they are at a loss to know what to do about it.

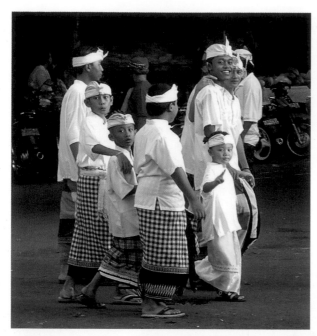
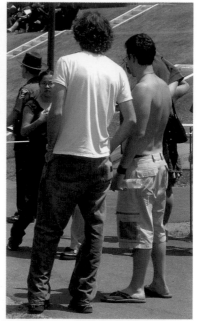
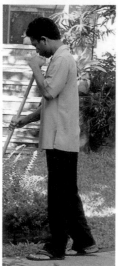
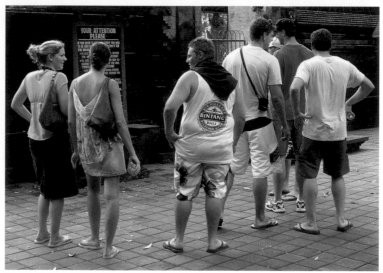

Comparison of these photos reveals that the contrast between still-aligned and no-longer-aligned children is not only evident between years past and the present but between children and young adults here in the United States and those who live in certain other places in the world.

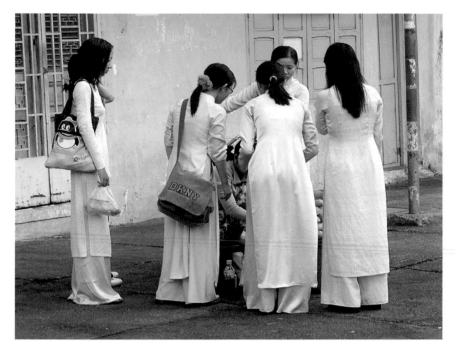

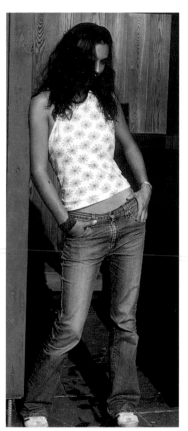

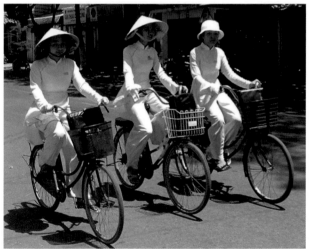

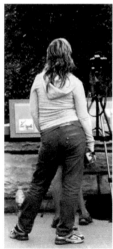

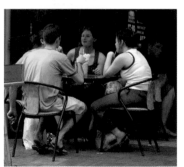

A relaxed, flowing quality is evident among these young Vietnamese girls who live in naturally aligned bodies. Their clothing hangs smoothly and evenly, giving them a graceful, flowing appearance that matches the symmetry of the skeletons that support them. Conversely, young people who are not aligned often take on a variety of shapes, none of which are natural. They may shift their weight back and forth between one leg and the other while standing, often with the fibers of their muscles and their clothing both askew.

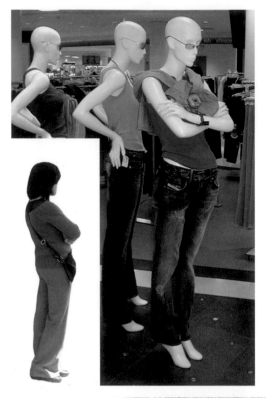

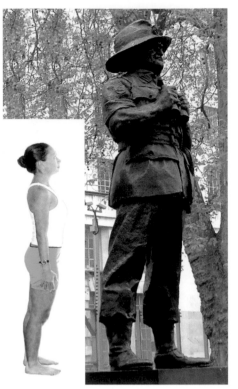

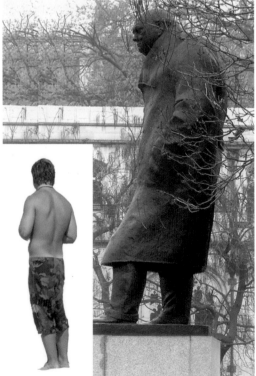

These photos exemplify how our children are subconsciously presented, on an almost daily basis, with examples of misaligned posture.

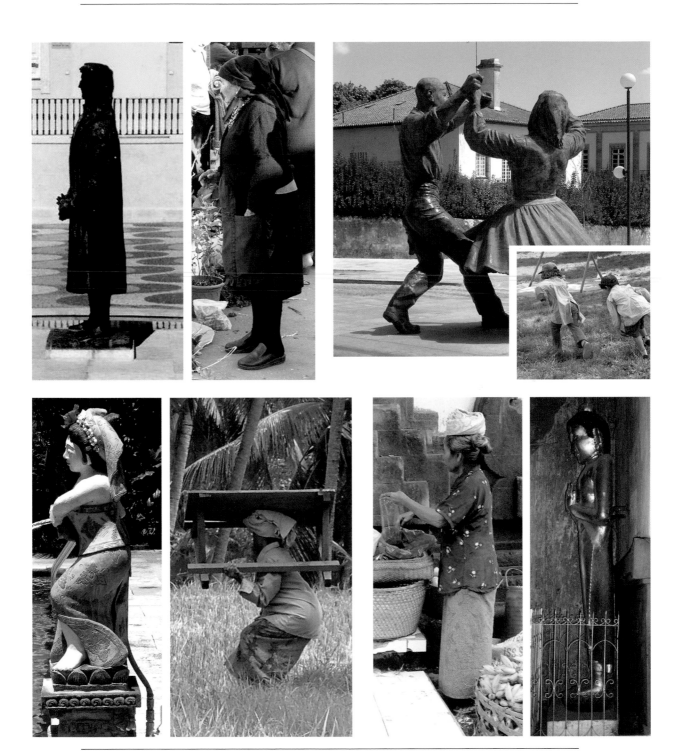

In some places in the world different examples predominate. Not surprisingly, a greater number of people in these places appear to reflect the natural alignment of the statues and icons in their environment.

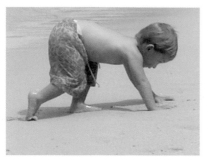
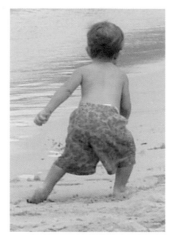
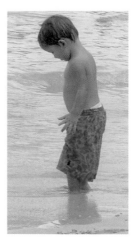
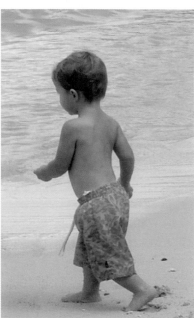
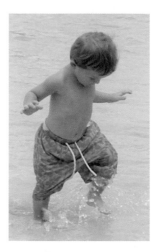
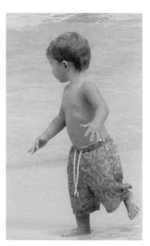

This little boy is a master of natural movement that reinforces an elongated spine in every move he makes. His movements are coordinated, strong, and dynamic. His playfulness at the beach models how the human body is designed to move with efficiency, comfort, and ease. Every action he takes maintains the integrity of his spine's alignment so that it is possible for him to be both relaxed and physically dynamic at the same time. No unnecessary muscular tension is called into play, only the minimum required to move the bones by bending at the appropriate joints. Anyone wanting to relearn how to move naturally could take lessons from this child and the many others like him.

The familiar adage "You're only as old as your spine" speaks to the fact that how we age is directly related to the condition of the spine. Clearly the adolescent girl and boy shown in the pictures on page 143 already have the spines, and perhaps some of the accompanying health problems, of very old, misaligned men and women.

One way we can support our children in remaining natural is in examining the part that certain role models or pop idols play and the messages that we regularly send our children. There may be some value in acknowledging that some of our cultural icons, both past and present, as great as we may believe they are, do not demonstrate the good posture that comes with relaxed, natural alignment. Over time, as our awareness of what natural alignment is and how important it is to our health and well-being, it may be that our icons themselves will begin to reflect the changes happening within us.

PROMISING THERAPIES TO COMBAT THE RISE OF AUTISM DISORDERS

Autism has been diagnosed with alarming frequency in recent years. Changes in the identification of various symptoms and the definition of shifting diagnoses may have contributed to the steep climb seen in recent years, but the scope of this epidemic remains nothing short of shocking, as the chart below so clearly reveals.

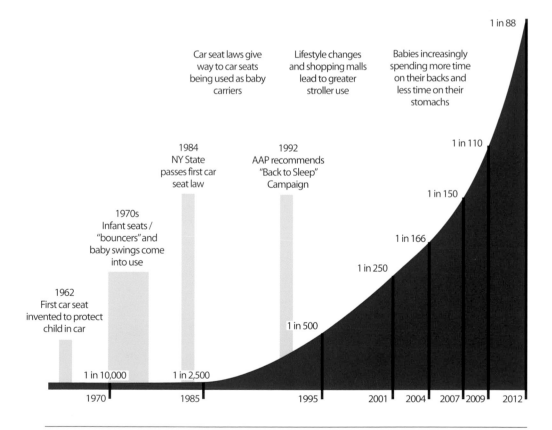

This graph charts the rise in autism over the past forty years.[8]

The numbers here only address autism, not ADHD or dyslexia or a collection of learning disabilities, childhood bipolar disorder, behavior problems, sleep disorders, eating disorders, vision problems, childhood depression, obsessive-compulsive disorder, Tourette's syndrome, chronic unexplained pain, or any of the epidemics affecting so many children today. No doubt there are a number of factors that play a role in these problems, but so far none has been investigated that provides anything that even approaches a clear answer.

Adding cultural trends such as the institution of car seat laws and the 1992 "Back to Sleep" campaign to the chart, while far from conclusive, raises questions that cannot be ignored. First and foremost is the question of infants spending more and more time on their backs, starting twenty years ago, and how this coincides with an astronomical increase in autism during this same period. When so many other factors have been investigated—including immunizations and environmental and dietary factors—that have not revealed a clear cause, we may be missing a significant piece of the puzzle by ignoring the growing pattern of structural collapse of the spine and nervous system that matches the skyrocketing incidence of neurodevelopmental disorders in children. Without adequate research it is impossible to say with any certainty if these are related.

Hippotherapy

New developments are now pointing toward promising results in the lives of a growing number of children, including those with autism and cerebral palsy, from participating in certain kinds of remedial physical activity.[9] This is occurring in instances where, whether by design or by happy accident, the body is brought closer to its natural alignment and development of core strength.

> Hippotherapy is a treatment approach used by trained therapists that utilizes activities on a horse to help patients improve in function, coordination, mobility, and balance. The term comes from the Greek *hippo*, which means "horse" and dates back, as a therapy, to the writings of Hippocrates.

Among those who have benefitted from hippotherapy is Temple Grandin, the most well-known and influential person to have struggled with and overcome some of the most debilitating aspects of autism. One of the major factors in Grandin's

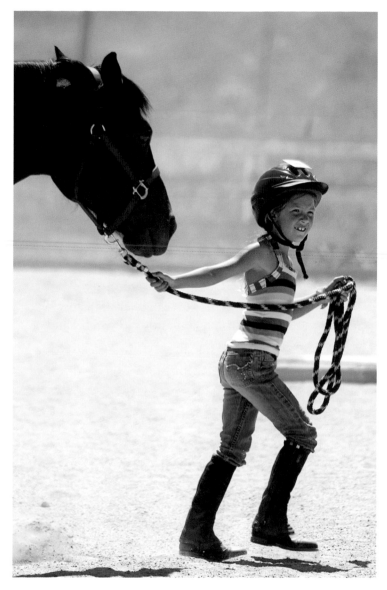

Key to the success of horseback riding in treating certain neurological disorders is the positioning of the pelvis and rib cage that strengthens the core.

journey to better health and improved functioning was her introduction to horseback riding.[10] Grandin has always had, as have others who face the challenges of autism spectrum disorders, a keen sense of kinship with animals and a profound sensitivity to their feelings.

Another detail that may have been overlooked as playing a part in the progress of Grandin and others is how the anteverted pelvis is reinforced while sitting on a saddle. This would help explain the growing number of children who are showing positive improvement of a host of symptoms after participating in therapeutic horseback riding programs.[11] As long as a forward rolling rib cage aligns with an anteverted pelvis, the entire spinal cord is open to a flow between body and brain that is tethered in place by a strong natural core. This appears to have been missing to varying degrees for some of these children. If someone were to ride a horse with a tucked under pelvis, the connection with the horse would be broken, and the ride would be bumpy, disjointed, and uncomfortable for both the rider and the horse. The combination of an anchored pelvis, a long, open spine, and feet and thighs connecting with the ground (the stirrups and horse's body) may be what it takes to not only connect the body with the brain but also the rider with the horse. I was able to witness the horse and rider connection in a profound way when working with an accomplished young rider named Sarah, who regularly experienced back pain when riding her horse.

As Sarah and her horse circled the perimeter of a riding pen in New Mexico, I stood in the center of the ring observing Sarah's riding posture. I could see that her pelvis was anchored solidly in the saddle, with her sitz bones out behind her and her pubic bone aiming down into the saddle—so far, so good. However, Sarah's

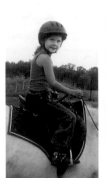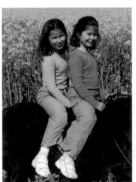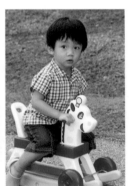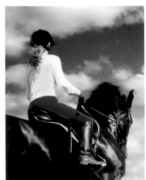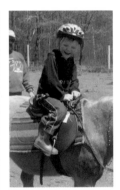

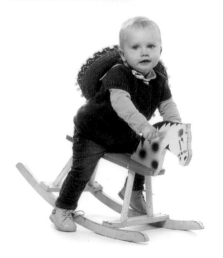

Riding a horse does not guarantee proper alignment, although straddling the width of the horse's middle encourages anteversion of the pelvis, shifting the body's weight over the front of it. This may explain why hippotherapy can be so effective in certain cases.

rib cage was rotated backward, with her chest lifted up in front, causing her back to arch and tighten, thus breaking her connection with the horse (or ground). At the precise moment when Sarah succeeded in dropping the front of her chest and releasing her lower back, her horse suddenly let out a long, dramatic whinny—perhaps a horse version of a sigh of relief.

A growing number of occupational therapists and physical therapists are becoming aware of the importance of core strength in children, although confusion about what real, bona-fide core strength actually is still continues.

Natural Movement as Occupational and Physical Therapy

While access to opportunities for riding horses is beyond the reach of many children, exciting developments similar to some of the best that hippotherapy has to offer are now being reported from a number of arenas, including a small town in New Jersey where, not long ago, a young woman named Daisy had a dramatic recovery after years of struggling with developmental difficulties. Daisy's symptoms, over the course of eighteen years, were variously identified and diagnosed as Asperger's syndrome, autism spectrum disorder, ADHD, and nonverbal learning disorder.

Although many therapies had been tried in an attempt to improve mood, emotional, social, and behavior performance, Daisy's mother finally came to the disappointing conclusion that her daughter continued to be "off" and that her needs were not being met by any of the approaches that had been applied. After enrolling her daughter in an intensive program of occupational and physical therapy for SPD (sensory processing disorder), Daisy's mother observed the most significant changes to date. As she evaluated these changes she began to notice, and then question, Daisy's long-standing postural collapse and low muscle tone.

With the assistance of an innovative yoga teacher in the community, Daisy's mother embarked on an informal study of yoga, principles of natural alignment, balance, and natural movement. Together they developed core exercises that stabilized an aligned spine and supported a well-functioning nervous system. Within a matter of months remarkable changes unfolded. Daisy's symptoms began to drop away, replaced by a quality of vibrancy, an engagement with others, and new, heightened competency. I recently met Daisy, a charming, intelligent, and well-spoken young woman who drove me around her community and told me about some of these changes and how her life has improved. She now looks forward to a bright future.* Her former principal and teachers and her family and neighbors have all been amazed at the transformation they have witnessed, leading some parents in the community to seek help with their own children from Daisy's mom and the yoga teacher. The results have been similar. Coincidence?

Is it simply a coincidence that, as more and more babies have lost the power of their core due to a chronically tucked-under pelvis, the incidence of neurological disorders has climbed through the roof? Without meaningful research it is impossible to know the answer to this, but one thing is crystal clear: until we begin to understand the body's natural human design and then examine how disruption of this design affects children's healthy development, we are guilty of a serious oversight.

WHAT CAN BE DONE

A growing number of occupational therapists, physical therapists, early childhood educators, chiropractors, hippotherapists, and body movement specialists have begun to recognize the value of greater physical involvement by children who are challenged in these ways. Children who struggle with symptoms of developmental disorders often share the same physical characteristics as Daisy—poor posture, low muscle tone, and dysfunctional movement patterns. Generally, children who appear perfectly healthy and normal at birth do not just suddenly develop neurodevelopmental symptoms for no reason. Nor do they end up with postural collapse or dysfunctional movement patterns, especially in ever-growing numbers, simply because of the luck of the draw. The fact that it is now being recognized that focused physical engagement is beneficial in helping to heal a variety of symptoms across the full panoply of neurodevelopmental disorders is a strong indication that we are moving in the right direction. In fact, in many cases there may be one common underlying cause: disruption of the natural human structural design. This appears to scramble, in one way or another, the transmission of signals between motor and sensory neurons and the brain, affecting the brain's ability to effectively interpret and act upon those signals. With neuroscientists intently focused on the

---

*Avigail Roberg and Miriam Krupinsky worked together to help Avigail's daughter, Daisy, reverse symptoms of autism spectrum disorder that had plagued her since early childhood. Now twenty years old, Daisy is a high-functioning, vibrant, and beautiful young woman. For more information refer to www.daisyorganization.com/index_files/humblebeginnings.htm.

most microscopic and complex details of brain function, it may turn out that a large piece of the puzzle is more simple than we've imagined and that we have overlooked the obvious.

Effectively addressing these problems is going to require greater curiosity and unorthodox thinking about how the human body actually works, as dictated by natural laws. We have to be willing to stretch our minds outside of the proverbial box that restricts our thinking to conditioned assumptions about things such as good posture, fitness, and conventional wisdom, all of which may not be entirely true. To do this we have to start looking beyond our own geographic borders to those places in the world where people inhabit bodies that move with ease through all the decades of a long lifetime. We have to study the healthy models, not just those with a dis*order* or a dis*ease,* two words that, when broken down, accurately describe their deeper meaning. Toddlers who have not yet lost the *orderliness* of an aligned skeleton, relatively small people who successfully carry heavy loads on their heads with *ease,* and people of an advanced age who maintain easy flexibility and elongated spines all hold the keys for showing us how to protect babies from losing their natural connection to good health. They also point the way back to the center and show us how to heal a broken connection that has already occurred.

Parents, teachers, physical education instructors, and sports coaches must all play a key role in turning these problems around. It will be the parents, like Daisy's mother, more than the educators and health professionals, who will drive a movement that demands that blinders be removed and new ways of looking for meaningful change be adopted. So far, there are few resources that offer tools for

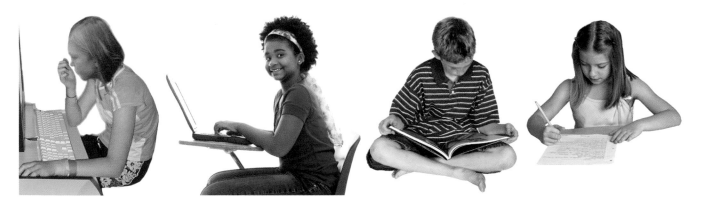

Most children spend hours each day, their spines curled and collapsed, sitting in front of television and computer screens. Added to this is the fact that the chairs they sit in, both at home and at school, and the height of the screen and the keyboard, often force them to sit in ways that only exacerbate the problem.

knowing how to do this. One of my earlier books, *Sad Dog Happy Dog: How Poor Posture Affects Your Child's Health & What You Can Do About It* (Mekevan Press, 2010) discusses steps that parents, teachers, and students can take, in a process of mutual learning, to make the shift from being sad or tense dogs to being happy dogs. Rather than this being incidental to a child's life, it should be central to their education when we understand the impact structural misalignment has on their health and well-being.

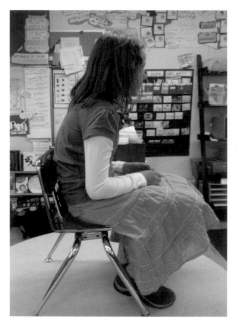 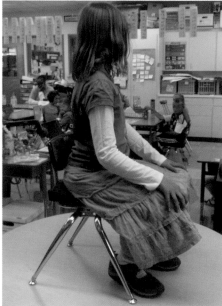 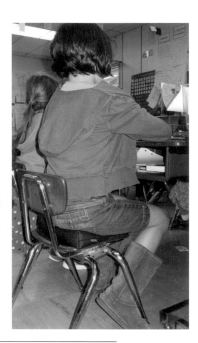

Use of a small wedge-shaped cushion that elevates the sitz bones is a helpful prop for sitting at a piano or desk, driving a car, or watching a movie or concert. Such a lift parks the pelvis in a happy dog position and supports an upright spine.

Parents and teachers can monitor how children are sitting and participating in various activities. In the same way that a parent would insist that a child not eat a sugary snack instead of a nutritious meal, a parent can also guide a child to understand the value of being a happy dog while watching a favorite television show, playing a video game, or reading a book. This must be done through positive encouragement, not judgment or blame, but parents are justified in insisting on this. Many of the images in this book can be useful for initiating a dialogue with children about the importance of natural alignment in their lives.

I have developed a small portable cushion, the Wedge, for just this purpose. (See resources for more details.) The Wedge is being used successfully in classrooms, and teachers whose students learn how to shift from being sad dogs to happy dogs report that their students are generally more settled and calm and focus better when sitting with a long, upright spine.

CHILDREN HEALING THEMSELVES

Most children respond enthusiastically when given the opportunity to get to know themselves as bodies. They are not only genuinely curious about how their bodies work, they are also grateful to be given permission to *feel* what is going on inside their skin. Even the most disengaged or overactive child will usually participate and listen when the conversation shifts to the life of the body. This is great news for parents, teachers, and health professionals, who can capitalize on children's interest by demonstrating that they too are interested in participating alongside their children in a process of mutual learning. Children are keenly sensitive to anything that resembles hypocrisy and respect us all the more when we demonstrate that we are willing to walk our talk.

Principles of natural alignment can be incorporated into the curriculum and daily life in the classroom. Ask a group of children how they feel, and you will discover that a remarkable number of them frequently experience pain while sitting at their desks or on the floor. It is impressive how often their pain is alleviated when they learn to rely on the support of naturally aligned bones. Once they directly experience the benefits of being happy dogs, with a pelvis that is able to support an easily upright spine, they grow in power over one of the most basic circumstances of their lives. Greater self-esteem and confidence is sure to grow from this as well.

It makes perfect sense that executive function, the part of the brain that acts as managing director and regulates the ability to organize thoughts and activities, would be enhanced by sharpening the mind's attention on the present moment. When we also incorporate the body into this process the benefits of this approach are multiplied. For one thing, an aligned skeleton allows all the body's systems, including respiratory, circulatory, and nervous system processes, to function at their highest level, able to deliver abundant supplies of oxygenated blood to the brain. An aligned spine becomes an open channel for billions of sensory and motor neurons

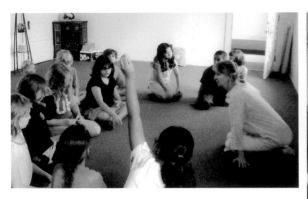

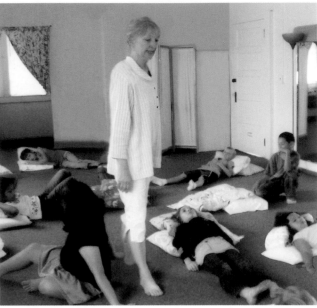

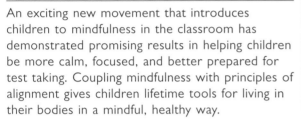

An exciting new movement that introduces children to mindfulness in the classroom has demonstrated promising results in helping children be more calm, focused, and better prepared for test taking. Coupling mindfulness with principles of alignment gives children lifetime tools for living in their bodies in a mindful, healthy way.

to transmit messages back and forth between the brain and the rest of the body. Awareness of the body itself becomes a solid, rooted anchor to the present moment that can perhaps be described best as embodied presence. Encouraging this awareness in children is a gift we give them that enhances their capacity for happiness and compassion, both now and in the future.[12]

Children whose skeletons are misaligned and whose muscles must work under strain at all times are ill equipped to participate in sports. They are put at great risk of suffering injuries. The alarming rise in sports injuries in children is blamed on what is now being called overuse syndrome, thought to result from playing one sport repetitively. The condition of a child's alignment when playing a sport is rarely considered to be a factor, yet physical activity that is repetitive and demanding is rarely a problem for children who remain naturally aligned. Children's bodies are still developing, and some of these injuries have serious implications, both now and into the future, such as osteoarthritis and repeated surgeries.

Until now, parents, educators, and health professionals have been at a loss to know what to do about children's worsening collapse—at home, in the classroom, and on the sports field. Repeated attempts to get children to sit or stand up "straight" have met with such continuous failure that the problem has begun to fall off the radar altogether.

Somewhat like the proverbial frog placed into a pot of slowly warming water, we are largely unaware of the shocking structural collapse that is occurring rou-

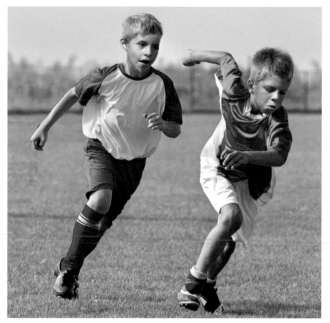

The boy on the left is moving easily from his core; his aligned structure is able to distribute the impact of GRF and forces of gravity throughout his body. The boy on the right, with his sad dog pelvis and collapsed core, has no core to stabilize his body while moving, leaving his joints at risk and making him vulnerable to pain and injury.

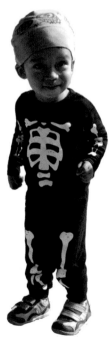

The balanced alignment of a child's skeleton is critical, and we must not lose sight of its importance.

tinely in more and more children, at younger and younger ages. Having lost a sense of what a wholly natural body looks like, most parents, teachers, and health professionals are unaware of the problem in the first place. The good news is that once the spotlight is shone on the problem, we can begin to acquire the tools needed to affect positive change.

7

AMAZING GRACE

CHANCES ARE GOOD that if you live in a technologically developed part of the world you will not run across many people of advanced age who have elongated spines like the ones pictured below.

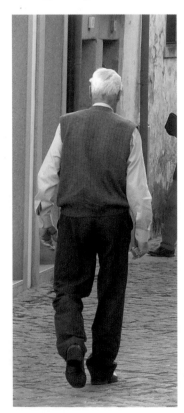

This man's age is unknown.

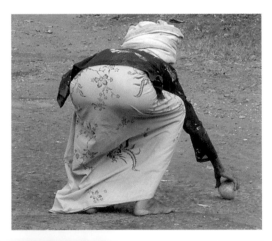

This woman is ninety-three years old.

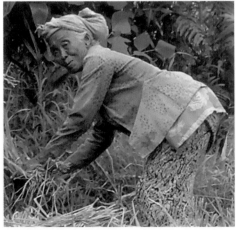

This woman is eighty-six years old.

In the same way that young children's bodies line up along the central axis, these people's bodies are divided almost perfectly in half by the axis many decades later. This is the potential that everyone comes into the world possessing.

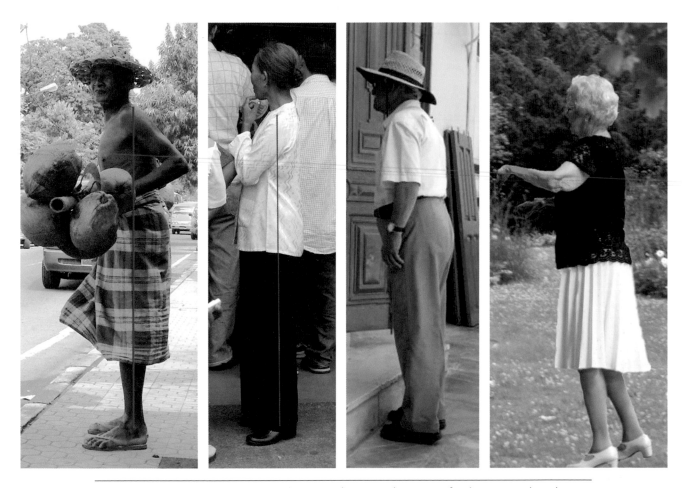

Note how the red line depicting the central axis is almost perfectly centered in the first two individuals. You can easily imagine such a line equally centered on the bodies of the two remaining individuals.

When we enter our later years with an optimally extended supple spine, the transition is likely to be less abrupt. While we will no doubt be slowing down, we are more likely to have relatively relaxed shoulders, flexible hips, lightness in our step, a natural store of energy, and fewer aches and pains.

Not long ago people thought that how one aged was simply the luck of the draw. Some people seemed to have all the luck and managed to move into old age still standing tall and feeling far more comfortable with their bodies. They may

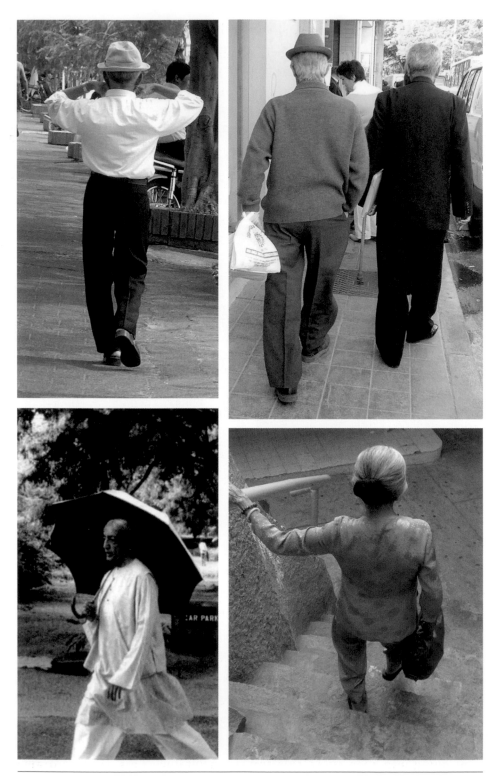

These people epitomize aging gracefully.

have found themselves stiffening up a little bit, but all in all their bodies didn't cause them a lot of problems. These people glided into old age more gently than those other folks who seemed doomed to be victims of gravity's commands, sinking into collapsed shapes that left them aching and stiff much of the time.

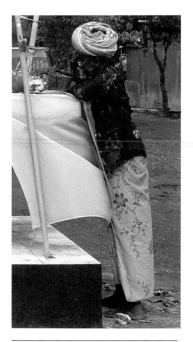

This woman is ninety-three years old.

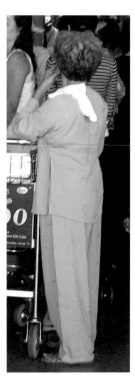

This woman's age is unknown.

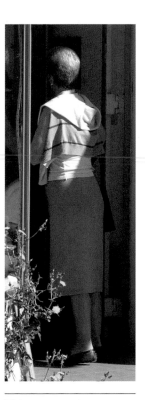

This woman is seventy-two years old.

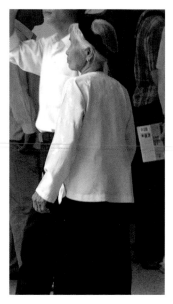

This woman is eighty-four years old.

In recent years studies have clearly determined that inactivity plays an important role in whether people age with greater ease. Use it or lose it has become the motto of the senior citizen exercise set; the relief many people feel when they become more active bears out what is true about this slogan. In the future, however, as research continues to examine what contributes to healthy aging, it is sure to come to light that how our skeletal structure is aligned in the first place may play an even bigger role in how we age than the degree to which we are active. In other words: *How you use it* is how you keep it!

We tend to think that images like those on the following pages represent typical aging and that aging this way is inevitable. This kind of dramatic structural collapse did not happen overnight. While it certainly is no one's fault

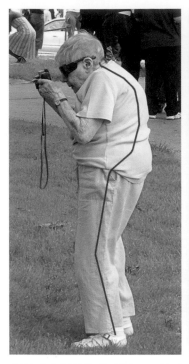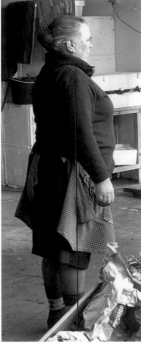

A comparison of these two women provides a dramatic example of how differently one can age depending on skeletal alignment.

that this occurred, this is the outcome of decades of tucking the butt.

People who have lived with aligned bones their whole lives enjoy a quality of *being* that is fluid, easeful, relaxed, free, comfortable, solid, capable, and accepting. Such people often take pleasure in remaining physically active well into old age. While certain economic realities often require that some people work longer, the concept of retirement appears to be both foreign and unwelcome to many who have aged with ease.

Certainly there are many things that happen in life that are beyond our control. How we age, however, is generally not one of them. Aging doesn't simply happen all of a sudden, nor is it simply the luck of the draw. The seeds are sown and the patterns are set into place (and our musculature) beginning at an early age.

It's never too late to apply principles of natural alignment and begin to improve our situation. Obviously change comes more slowly the older we are, and the level of change that is possible becomes more difficult. This is why it is so important for us to protect children from never losing their natural alignment in the first place and to resolve misalignment as early as possible.

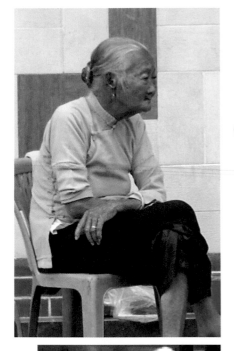

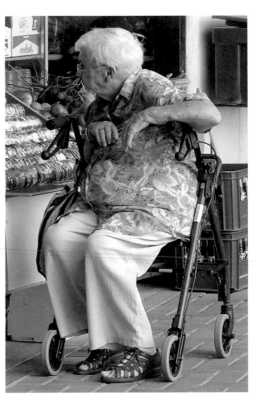

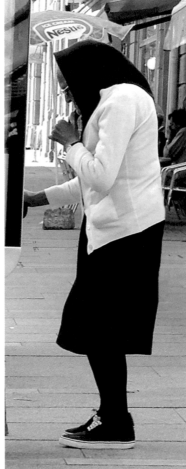

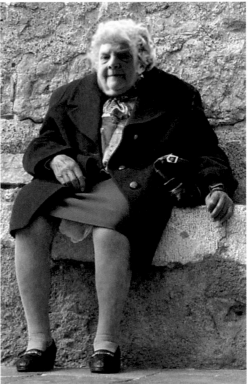

Without the support of aligned bones, skeletal collapse defines aging.

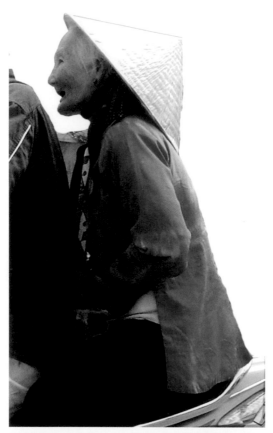

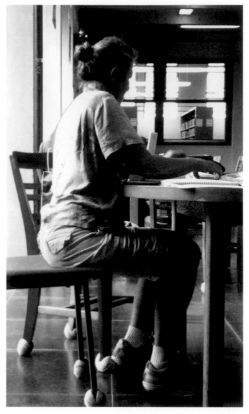

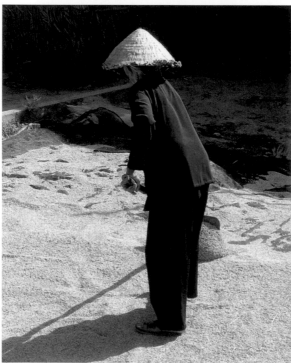

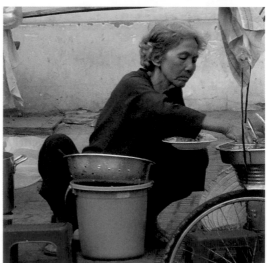

An aligned core provides us with the ability to continue being physically active during old age.

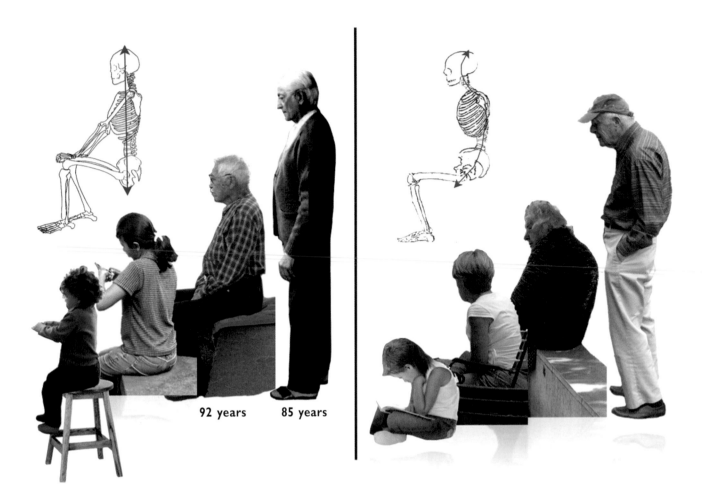

92 years   85 years

Looking at the skeletons pictured above, it's not difficult to see how, when bones are perpetually out of alignment, over and over again, when we are sitting, standing, and walking, bending and lifting—even sleeping—that the muscles attached to those bones take on an unnatural length and hold the bones out of alignment.

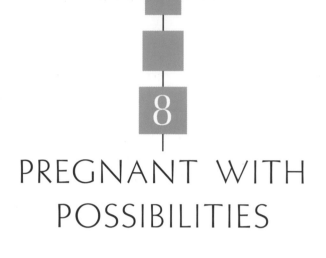

8

PREGNANT WITH POSSIBILITIES

PREGNANCY IS A TIME of great change; the body of the mother-to-be swells with the growth of life within her. It can be a time of great excitement and antici-pation that can also present a woman with new challenges she has not faced before. Among these is finding ease and comfort in her body over the months of physical changes that make room for a growing baby and the inevitable demands this places on her body. It is not uncommon for expectant mothers to experience back pain, sciatica, heartburn, swollen ankles, and insomnia to one degree or another. For some women these problems can be particularly difficult.

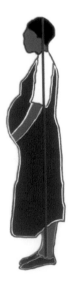

Most women do not realize that many of these problems can be alleviated, at least in part, by using the body's natural design to support the many changes to her body over the coming months.

Pregnancy and childbirth are as natural to humans as to all other species. It is easy to forget this in the modern world of scheduled cesarean deliveries, fetal-heart monitors, epidurals, fluorescent-lit nurseries, and baby bottles. Babies are more likely to thrive when they are born to a mother who has taken good care of herself over the previous months and who is comfortable and relaxed with what is happening to her. Chances are good that a woman who is relaxed and comfortable during her pregnancy will be more likely to have an uncomplicated delivery and move into motherhood with greater ease. Among other things, this requires self-awareness and a healthy body that conforms to its natural design. Few occasions offer a woman a greater opportunity to turn her attention inside her skin as she shares the months of her pregnancy with the small being growing inside her.

As the baby grows bigger within the uterus, the weight that is added on to the front of the mother-to-be has the potential to throw her off balance, especially if her bones are not aligned to begin with, which is, sadly, the case with so many expectant mothers today. This misalignment causes their center of gravity to be somewhat higher, causing them to have to lean backward above the waist as the baby grows larger in the front. This causes the spine to be compressed and puts tremendous stress on the lower back. Not only does this frequently cause back pain, it can also affect the easy flow of blood, lymph, and other fluids that are not only important for the mother's health and comfort but for that of the baby as well. Fortunately, a soon-to-be mother can learn how to counteract this tendency by applying basic principles of alignment that may save her back and allow her to have a far more enjoyable pregnancy.

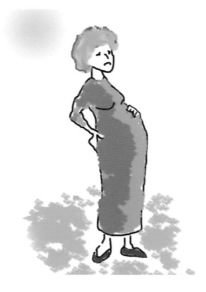

Not only is the back put at risk by the typical pregnant stance, but internal organs that are already crowded by the growing fetus can become even more compressed by faulty posture. This can lead to a whole host of digestive problems, shortness of breath, and fatigue.

A pregnant woman can learn how to call upon her inherent skeletal alignment and deep core of internal support to do the work of holding her up in a way that is comfortable and gives relief from many of the most common problems women experience, especially during the most challenging last months of pregnancy. When her bones are aligned, the core muscles actually function like a hammock that cradles the baby from below and helps hold baby and belly in place.

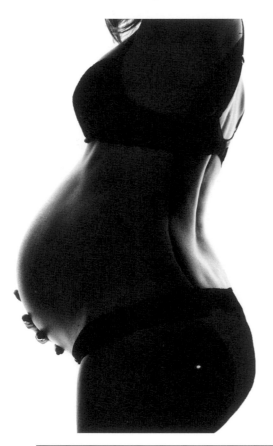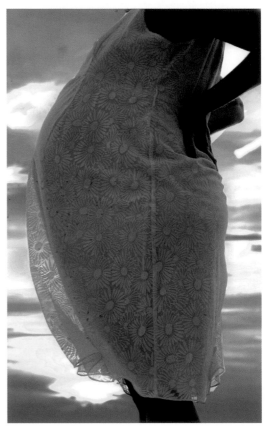

It has become common for a mother-to-be to be displaced forward of the axis, just at a time when she needs her body's inherent support more than ever. Excessive arching of the lower back (lordosis) and an opposite rounding of the upper back (kyphosis) can be the cause of back pain, restricted blood flow, and impingement on the diaphragm and its ability to function most efficiently.

The body of a pregnant woman should line up along the vertical axis. This allows the baby to fit compactly into the uterus, held in place by firm, elastic muscles. The mother's back should be long and open, not arched and tight. Holding the belly out to the front, forward of the axis, is the primary cause of the back pain so many pregnant women experience. This also gives many pregnant women a shape that is not that of a naturally ripening pregnant belly but the shape of a larger-than-natural, ballooning belly that is often characteristic of a host of stresses pregnant women experience.

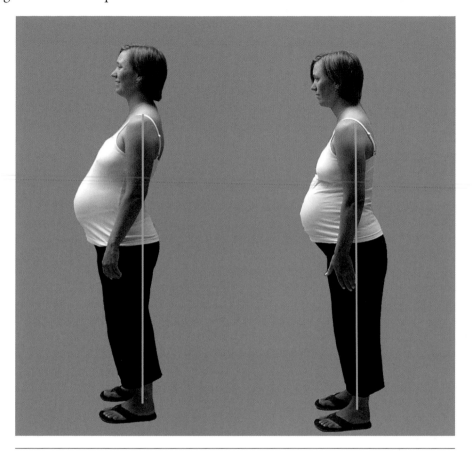

On the left, this woman's skeleton is forward of the axis, pushing her belly, and the baby, out in front of her. On the right, she is in the proper, aligned stance that is best for mother and baby.

Sitting in a natural position becomes doubly important for the woman who carries an almost full-term baby in her belly. When she sits without the direct support of her sitz bones but, instead, with her pelvis tilted backward her torso collapses throughout. Gravity bears downward, pushing the weight of the fetus, placenta, and amniotic fluids onto the mother's internal organs. Breathing is somewhat restricted when the diaphragm gets pinched and crowded in this position. It is not difficult to understand why pregnant women complain so often of back pain, heartburn, constipation, fluid retention, and shortness of breath. However, the mother-to-be who sits on her sitz bones and lets her spine support her torso is far less likely to experience these difficulties. It is not difficult to see why, because the baby is supported from below by the cross fibers of the transversus abdominis and oblique muscles and does not push down on the mother's organs from above.

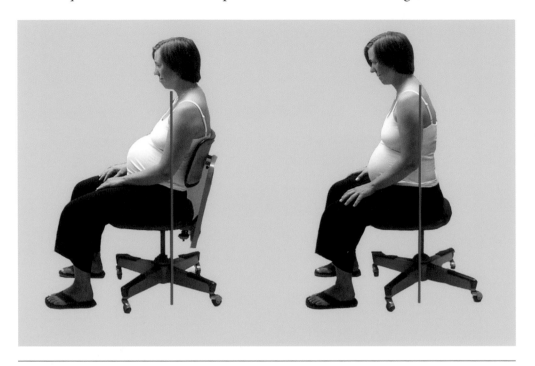

Sitting back on the pelvis as shown on the left is likely to cause much discomfort as the weight of the baby is not properly supported. Sitting as shown on the right is good practice for keeping the floor of the pelvis open and relaxed, which will be an important detail during the birthing of her baby.

Knowing how to sit, stand, and bend is important for anyone but most especially so for the woman who is actively moving for two. By taking her cue from toddlers who demonstrate how to move in an easy and natural way, she will greatly enhance her ability to enjoy her time being pregnant. In addition, knowing which comfortable positions she can take for sleeping and resting will provide her with ways to practice the important art of relaxing in preparation for the big day.

Preparation for labor and delivery is greatly enhanced by knowing how to sit and squat in natural ways and how to release the pelvic floor. These are made possible by having the pelvis in the natural anteverted position throughout the whole pregnancy. Most of all, those same deep core muscles that have supported the baby in the womb will now come into play to bear down and move the baby through an open, aligned birth canal.

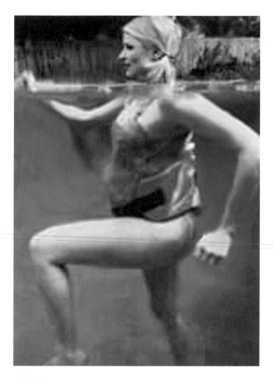

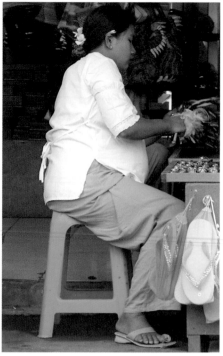

This woman prepares for the birth of her child by exercising with an aligned core.

Moving and sitting in a relaxed and natural way, with an anteverted pelvis, throughout her pregnancy will likely help this woman when it is time to give birth.

A laboring woman's ability to relax greatly increases her chances for having a natural birth, the best kind of experience for her and her baby.

Perhaps nothing interferes more with the natural process of a baby being born than the mother's body having to work against its natural design. A backward-tilted pelvis tightens all the wrong muscles and interferes with the ability of the core muscles to help push the baby out. Instead of the body being set up to open and release, all the messages it is getting are about closing up and holding on. For this reason any exercises done during pregnancy should adhere to the basic principles of natural alignment and emphasize both the core that will give the baby a boost on its way into the world and the mother's ability to "line up all the parts" and then relax and allow it all to happen.

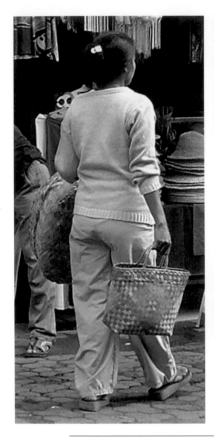
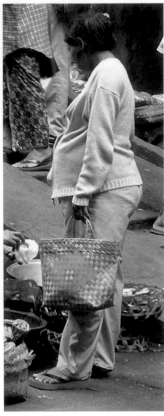
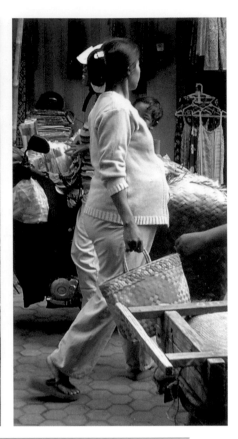

From behind it is impossible to tell that this young woman is pregnant, because she is so aligned and relaxed and moves with such ease. Pregnancy comes easily to her because she has lived in a naturally aligned body her entire life. Adjusting to the new demands of pregnancy appears to be easy for her. Without ever having to think about it, her bones support her and her baby. Her baby is also neatly cradled in place, tethered by elastic muscles, so she does not have to lean her upper body back in order to compensate for the added weight in front. Viewed from the side, this woman is seen to be quite far along in her pregnancy. A return to her normal state after the baby's birth will probably be accelerated by the ease with which she has moved through this pregnancy.

A physically easeful pregnancy sets the stage for a complication-free delivery. A mother-to-be who is not overcome by back pain, heartburn, and fatigue throughout her pregnancy is far more likely to have a birth experience for herself and her baby that reflects the ease with which she moved through the preceding nine months. Certainly, some complications occur that are beyond anyone's control. Nevertheless, many problems can be avoided when a woman conforms to and reinforces how her body is constructed to reproduce the same natural labor and delivery experienced by billions of mothers and babies throughout the ages.

POSTPARTUM NOTES

For all the relief and unbounded joy that often comes from finally having her baby in her arms, a new mother faces many other new challenges. One of these is how to comfortably lift and carry the baby, who only gets heavier with each passing day. Baby carriers that allow a mother or father to "wear" their baby come in handy at this stage and are of great benefit to parents and babies alike.

Breastfeeding, for all its many advantages, is very time consuming and can be a trying experience for a new mother if her back and neck are aching and tense. Knowing how to use her bones and her core muscles to help with lifting and holding the baby will greatly enhance the experience for everyone.

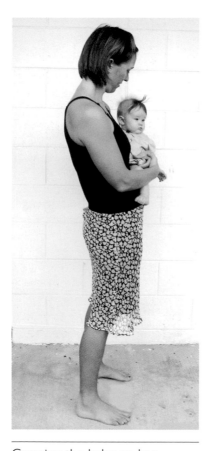

Carrying the baby on her hip while leaning back causes this mother to move out of alignment and will soon become uncomfortable.

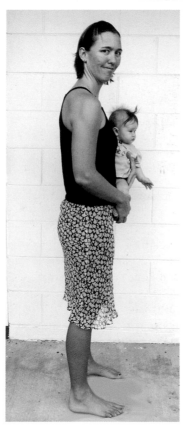

By holding her baby close to her body and remaining in an aligned stance, this new mother will have a much more enjoyable experience, greatly reducing the potential for neck and back pain.

Approximately 30 percent of women experience a condition called *diastasis recti,* a separation of the rectus abdominis muscle, the most superficial of the four layers of abdominal muscles[1] discussed in greater detail in chapter 3. Connecting the two sides of this muscle is a thick, fibrous band called the *linea alba,* which runs vertically from the xyphoid process at the base of the sternum to the pubis symphysis. This band becomes overstretched in some women, especially those with a posteriorly tilted rib cage, as the baby grows and the uterus pushes against the muscle, leading to weakness in the abdominal wall postpartum.

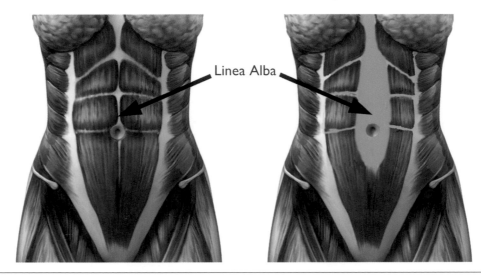

Linea Alba

The linea alba runs down the center of the abdomen from the xyphoid process to the pubis symphisis.

With time, the overstretched rectus abdominis muscle can be repaired, not by exercising it directly, but by strengthening the deeper transversus abdominis. As this muscle firms up in tone, its horizontal fibers have the effect of cinching the waist, like tightening a deeply internal belt or drawing together the strings on a purse. For this reason the trans ab could also be called the

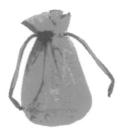

As the transversus abdominis firms up, it tightens the waist like the drawstring on this purse.

"slimming muscle" with extra benefits for any and all women concerned about a widening waist.

Diastasis recti is yet another area waiting to be studied, and it would not be surprising to discover that this condition is far less prevalent in rural places in the world where childbearing women typically remain more aligned and supported by a stable core. Women's bodies are designed to withstand the rigors of a normal pregnancy, and while there are certainly exceptions to this, diastasis recti appears to be more common than it should be.

9

IN FITNESS OR IN HEALTH?

IT IS A FAIRLY RECENT concept that exercise, in order to be beneficial, must be performed almost to the point of exhaustion. No longer is it just those aspiring to be Olympians and super athletes who push themselves to the limit and beyond. Today many people of the twenty-four-hour fitness, no pain, no gain, set are convinced that sculpting and molding a body—creating the body you always wanted—will not only make them more attractive according to a culturally established ideal, but also will guarantee good health and longevity.

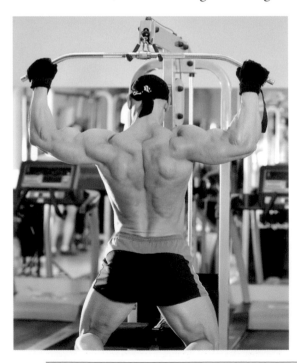 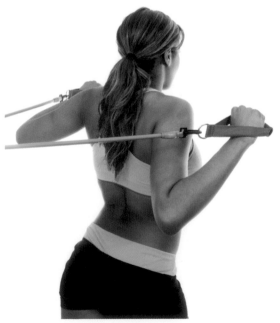

Creating a sculpted body is thought by many to be the path to good health.

Exercise has many obvious benefits: it burns calories, reduces body fat, lowers blood pressure, combats depression, increases bone density, and detoxifies the body, among other good things. For all these features exercise is also responsible for millions of injuries each year that include bulging or herniated discs, sciatica, rotator cuff injuries, torn ligaments, joint impingement, bursitis and tendonitis, and strains and sprains, to name only some of the problems.[1] Exercise, for some people, results in chronic pain and orthopedic surgeries such as hip and knee repair or replacement.

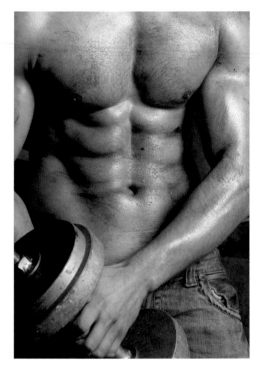

The hazards of exercise may not be immediately apparent but are very real.

One reason for the general failure to recognize the dangers associated with intensive working out is that exercise often feels good. Endorphins, those morphinelike polypeptides produced within the brain that reduce stress and relieve pain, bring a euphoric high to many people when they are released during exercise. This matches the sense of relief many people experience when exercising releases the tensions stored up in tight muscles. What many people don't realize is that they can become psychologically addicted to these feelings,[2] along with a need to repeatedly sweat or stretch away tensions that would not have accumulated in the first place if their bones were simply aligned. With aligned bones, muscles can remain relaxed and free from tension.

Building bulk into muscles draws the ends of bones closer together and compresses the joints, limiting their natural range of motion. This causes deterioration of cartilage and contributes to chronic shortening of the spine, herniation of discs, pressure on nerve roots, and strains and tears to soft tissue.

Pain and injuries are usually blamed on insufficient stretching and warming up before exercising, but, in most instances, this is not the real culprit. Most insidious among the hazards of many exercise routines is the persistent reinforcing of structural distortions such as the repeated shortening of the spine and compression of joints that go unnoticed until some point in the future when the impingement or pressure is too great on a joint or gravity deals a blow to a misaligned body that is unprepared to match its force. Unless one understands how to align the bones while engaging in exercise of any sort, short-term benefits will eventually be trumped by artificial patterns of movement that, in the long run, will do more harm than good. This is one of the primary reasons many people end up with chronic stiffness and pain and diagnoses such as osteoarthritis, spinal stenosis, and degenerative disc disease.

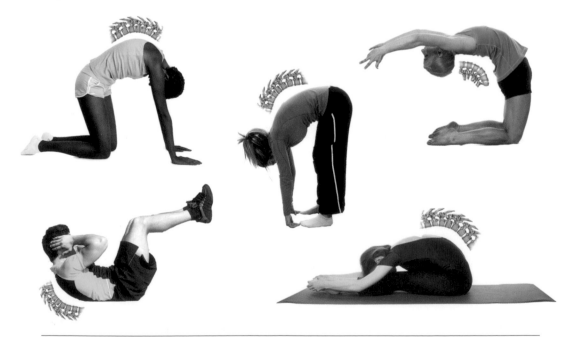

Stretching, done improperly, can be detrimental to our future health by destabilizing joints and building unnatural ways of moving.

For all the health benefits that are touted about getting enough exercise, little or no emphasis is placed on the crucial aspects of maintaining the body's *actual* natural alignment. When alignment or "good" posture is talked about, it is largely based on the myth of suck and tuck (suck in the belly and tuck the tail), the basic misunderstanding about good posture that causes fitness to dwell on the surface of the body—in muscles that can be seen as being ripped due to their pronounced shape and definition. A truly healthy body is bone deep and can be difficult to recognize or, for many people, difficult to accept because of conditioned beliefs about what fitness and attractiveness are supposed to look like.

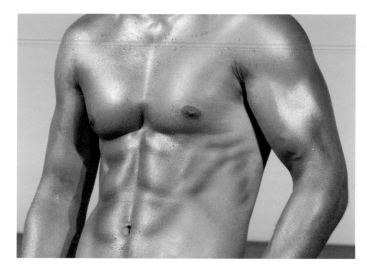

Most of us don't realize that the perception of what constitutes fitness and attractiveness has been trained into us.

Our society's recent and growing obsession with a type of fitness that goes *beyond* normal good health is a fairly recent phenomenon in the hundreds of thousands of years of human existence.

True fitness and health are not only our natural state, they define everything about how we live and move and how all the working parts and systems of the body function together as one integrated whole.

It can be difficult to accept the notion that exercise, in order to be beneficial, does not have to involve effort and struggle; especially when no pain, no gain has been a regularly repeated motto. T'ai chi, qigong, and aikido are among those forms of movement that lend themselves well to retraining the body back to its natural home base of alignment. These disciplines place an emphasis on awareness, breathing, movement of energy, and the body's natural alignment; this is the basis of their success over so many years.

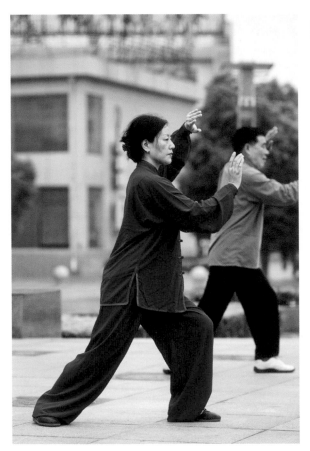

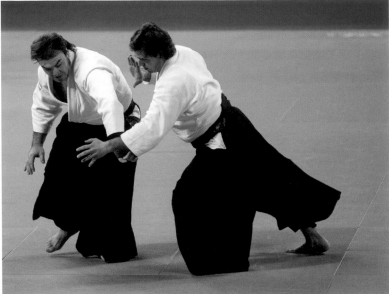

The most beneficial forms of exercise are those that work with the body, not against it, by reinforcing the most economical and efficient ways of moving. Inhabiting the body in this natural way is the best kind of anti-aging medicine that is available.

Martial arts training usually involves the development of qualities such as "undoing," nonresistance, relinquishing, and acceptance. Far from being easy to do, these practices require tremendous concentration and presence and carefully controlled movements that are initiated from a deep core (*tan tien,* meaning "energy core," or *hara,* meaning "belly" or "center of life"), along with adherence to the rules that govern the body's mechanical design. The strength one is able to make use of here is not a strength that is understood just by muscles. The strength that an aikido master calls forth is an extension of what is known as *ki,* or life force energy, a quality of being that is not so much cultivated as it is made manifest through a practice of aligning oneself with the truth of who we already are.

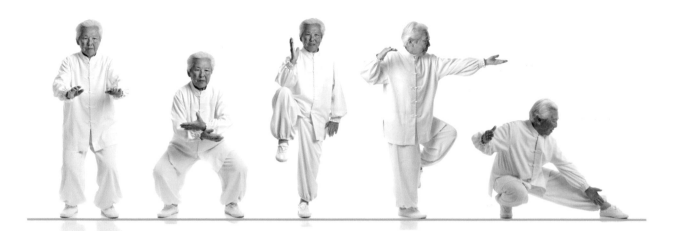

The fluidity and strength that comes from ki energy relies on skeletal alignment along the axis, essential to open channels through which the ki can move. Again and again this has been the overlooked feature that makes this innate energy available to all healthy humans, in the same way it is to this seventy-six-year-old woman.

Yoga, when practiced from a place of alignment, offers many benefits. Unfortunately, like any other activity, it is harmful when done with a body that is misaligned; entrenching poor habits of mechanical use, at best, and leading to injury and chronic pain, at worst. Perhaps the most common mistake that is made when practicing yoga is lifting up the chest (backward rotation of rib cage) and arching the back. This compresses the vertebrae and discs of the spine and creates tension in muscles of the neck and back.

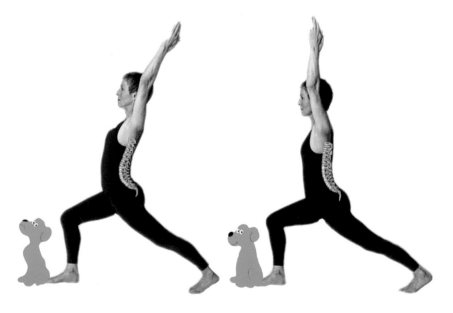

The image on the left is in a tense dog stance, greatly arching the spine. In the image on the right, the pelvis and rib cage relationship is intact, tethered in place by an engaged core. This allows for stability of the spine as it climbs up the back.

Because of the widespread popularity of yoga today, as well as the potential for injury and pain, chapter 12 ("Yoga on the Axis") addresses ways to practice yoga safely, so that it becomes more than just a way to relieve constant tension but a way to transform it so that stretching becomes less and less necessary to feeling relaxed.

TRADITIONAL DANCE AS AN EXPRESSION OF ALIGNMENT

Traditional dance has been a vital part of many cultures which have passed along, from one generation to the next, specific movements that are the basis of their particular style of dance.

More recent and independent styles of dance, which include ballet, modern dance, jazz, and hip hop are sometimes done in ways that cause unnatural distortions of the spine and joints, which can be problematic for the dancers' bodies. In some instances, one can imagine lifting the chest, particularly that of a solo dancer such as a prima donna, as being a physical assertion of the ego. (See chapter 10.)

The most flowing, agile dancers in the ballroom, swing, tango, salsa, and samba competitions, are the ones whose bodies remain aligned along the axis, their deep connection with the ground allowing them to be light on their feet, smooth in all their moves, and, like all naturally aligned athletes, least likely to suffer injuries and pain. Among the styles of dance that preserve this connection is *hula kahiko,* a traditional Hawaiian dance form that epitomizes the remarkable power and grace available through the human body's connection with the earth.

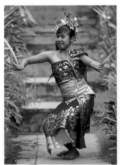 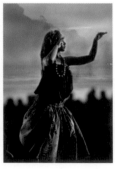 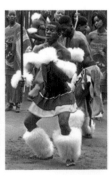 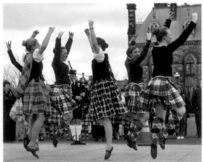 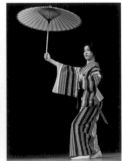

Characteristic of the sampling of ethnic dances pictured here—Balinese, Hawaiian, Zulu, Scottish, and Japanese—is an elongated spine that is supported by an anchored pelvis. The knees bend wide, the tailbone never tucks, and the feet connect deeply with, or push off deeply from, the earth. This draws up energy that fuels these aligned movements.

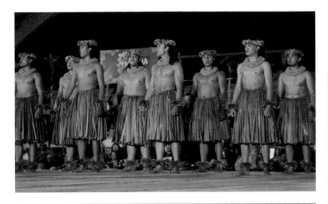

The legs of the men pictured here serve as conduits for an exchange of *mana,* the life force that moves through their bodies in an equal balance of strength and power that is matched with fluidity and ease of movement.

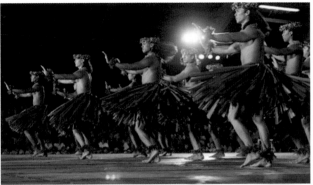

Notable among the ways that hula, when practiced naturally, reinforces the body's design are healthy, agile feet that engage deeply with the earth, a pelvis that is anchored in the natural anteverted position, a rib cage that remains tethered in place by natural core strength, and an elongated spine that is never displaced during the movements.

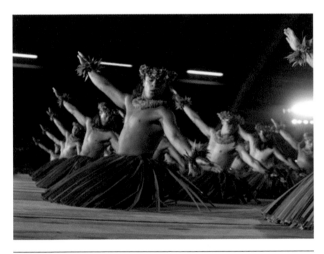

While these men all possess tremendous strength, their muscles are not overdeveloped in an unnatural way. This allows the deepest core strength to provide stability in everything they do. This includes keeping the integrity of the spine intact while performing the difficult maneuver of bending back to the floor while on their knees.

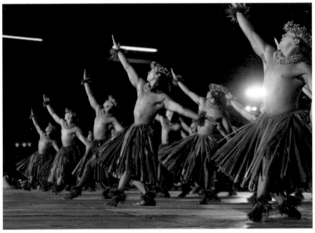

These superbly trained dancers of Halau i ka Wekiu reveal the true majesty of the human body that is available when we align with the axis and move from the core. Traditional Hawaiian culture, through dance, song, and chant, has always recognized and revered this profound human connection with the natural world.

IT'S QUITE A STRETCH

Actively stretching muscles has grown in popularity in recent years. Stretching is generally understood as being necessary for overall free movement. Unfortunately, stretching from a place of misalignment is done at the expense of an elongated spine, as seen below, and often ends up being an assault on tight muscles. Much of what is driving the recent popularity of stretching is how good it feels—stretching brings welcome relief from stiffness and tension that is stored in muscles. The kind of flexibility one gains from stretching, however, is not genuine and must be repeated on a regular basis. If the stretching is stopped, and the bones are not aligned, the tension and stiffness will always return. The place from which to start true healing—returning to the natural state—begins with aligning the bones.

Natural flexibility is always available as a by-product of living in a body that is structurally aligned. Muscles that are attached to aligned bones are inherently

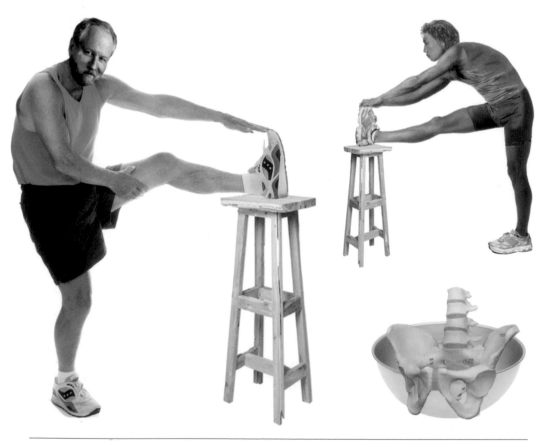

Bending to stretch from an unmoving pelvis causes shortening and compression in the front of the spine.

flexible, free of tension, and able to do their primary job of moving bones without effort or strain. This concept runs counter to many messages related to health and fitness in our culture, but a look at the men pictured here reveals an easy flexibility that is only possible from the natural, dynamic interplay between *aligned* bones and *elastic* muscles. Such flexibility is never regained in a lasting way by stretching but, instead, comes from promoting free range of motion in joints by moving naturally in all that we do, all day long.

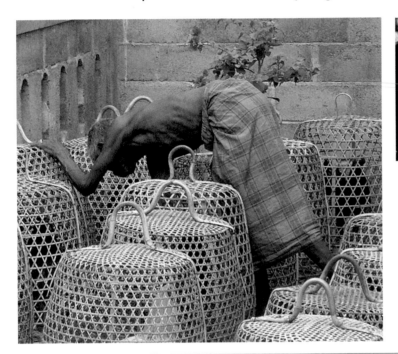

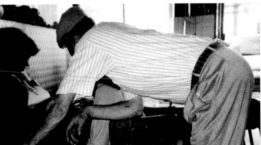

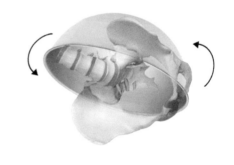

When bending is initiated by rotating the pelvis forward at the hip socket, with the spine remaining elongated and free of compression, strength in the core stabilizes and protects this "trunk of the tree."

Bending involves the sitz bones moving back as the pelvis rotates over the head of the femur (thighbone). The angle of the hip crease at the top of the leg closes to the degree to which the pelvis tips. Truly dynamic bending is initiated deep within an active core as the back of the rib cage rises upward. This engages GRF and gives the sense that, as the body engages down it is being "poured" up through the back and neck and out the top of the head.

Key to natural bending is the stability of the spine throughout the movement. This is tricky for many people who are conditioned to bend by lifting the chin and chest. This arches the lower back (extension of the spine) or, conversely, rounds the

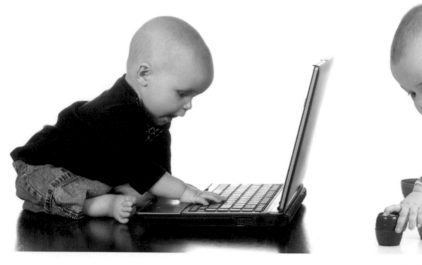

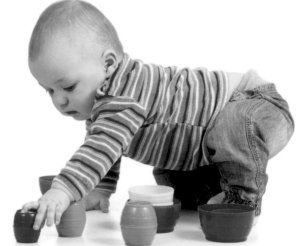

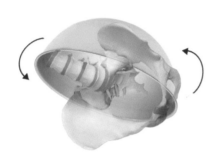

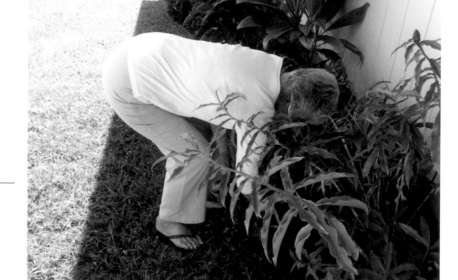

Notice that each of these individuals, babies and the 80-year-old woman, are bending by rotating the pelvis and not curving the back.

back when bending with a fixed, unmoving pelvis (flexion of the spine). Both of these are unnatural ways of bending and often lead to cumulative spinal problems in the long run. The use of the term *extension* has been co-opted by its current popular usage that refers to unnatural arching of the spine. For this reason it is helpful to keep in mind that what we are aiming to do, when bending forward and returning to an upright position, is keep the spine elongated. We do this by engaging the power button and stabilizing the spine.

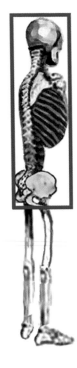
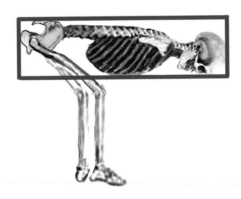

When bending, the goal is to begin in the position on the left and end in the position on the right. Notice that the spine is elongated at all times.

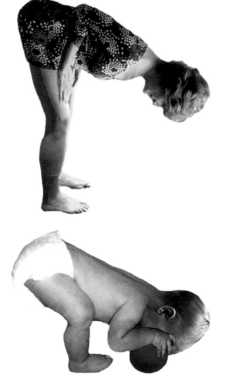
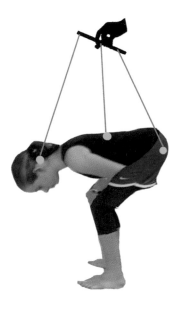

Notice how all three of these individuals maintain a straight spine that neither arches nor bends.

> In any given moment we are either elongating and opening the spine or shortening and compressing it. For this reason we must be mindful of our position and strive to elongate the spine.

FITNESS VS. HEALTH

The meaning of the word *fitness* needs to be refined to include an underlying quality of health made possible because of:

- an optimally elongated spine
- a solidly anchored pelvis
- a core of stability at the deepest level
- relaxed, natural breathing
- elastic superficial muscles free from excess tension
- a capacity to deeply relax
- open, free-moving joints

With all these qualities intact, true fitness would look like the people in the photos on the facing page.

Confusion exists among linguists over the definition of fitness, with some defining it as possessing a quality of overall health, while others emphasize a quality of developed strength through exercise. With the proliferation of so many gyms and health clubs and new ways of gauging stamina and muscle tone, fitness today appears to be focused primarily on the measurement of one's functional capacity to accomplish certain goals.

Health, on the other hand, reflects far more than just an absence of disease. It is an underlying quality of the entire organism that suggests a heart that functions well, with blood flowing freely through unrestricted blood vessels; breathing that is smooth and efficient; a nervous system that regularly restores itself in the parasympathetic mode and efficiently transmits messages to and from the brain; and an overall condition of the body that is not likely to succumb to disease any time soon. In spite of whatever contributions currently defined physical fitness does make in promoting good health, it promises none of these things. In fact, fitness, when defined as performance ability, does not even require that the body actually be in good health.

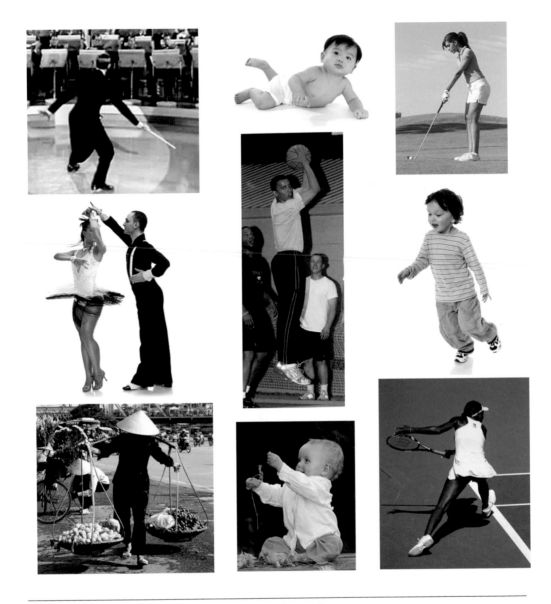

These people exemplify all of the qualities of true fitness.

People who enjoy running, playing sports, dancing, working out at the gym, practicing yoga or Pilates, and riding a bicycle should continue to freely enjoy these activities. The more the basic concepts of natural alignment are understood and put into practice, the more beneficial these activities will be. Those who despise formal exercise can probably take heart; although being a confirmed couch potato or sitting in front of a computer all day are not healthy options, in the same way that eating poorly has proven to be unhealthy. Everyone needs regular movement

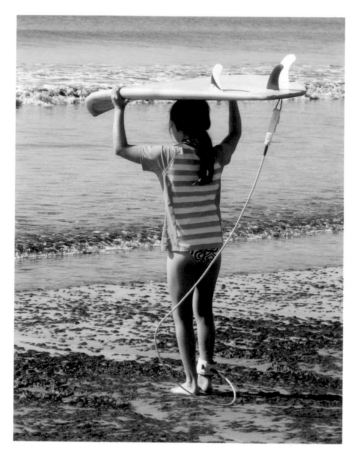

This girl might be considered fit simply because she has the physical ability to be a surfer. However, there is much more to true health and fitness than the ability to perform an athletic activity.

or some form of exercise to stimulate circulation and maintain normal, healthy stamina. Movement does not need to be excessive, however, and can easily include weeding the garden, washing windows, or walking around the neighborhood. The emphasis on a high level of daily exercise may one day be revised as new information about how structural alignment and active engagement with GRF reinforces healthy functioning of the heart and all the body's systems. The bottom line appears to be this: the only exercise worth doing is that which works *with* the body's design, not against it.

An aligned and balanced body does not need either extreme strength or flexibility, having more than enough of each to function in activities of normal daily living. This natural strength and flexibility can be maintained through living a normally active life well into old age.

The human body is a complex system made up of a number of smaller interdependent systems. When everything is working together as intended by the design of these systems, the result is a normal state of homeostasis, or balance. Central to good health is the ability of all the working parts and systems of the body to be able to function efficiently. The bare bones skeleton is the framework of support for each one of those systems, providing the structure within which internal organs, blood vessels, nerve cells, muscle fibers, and the flowing breath all coexist in a working partnership on behalf of the organism.

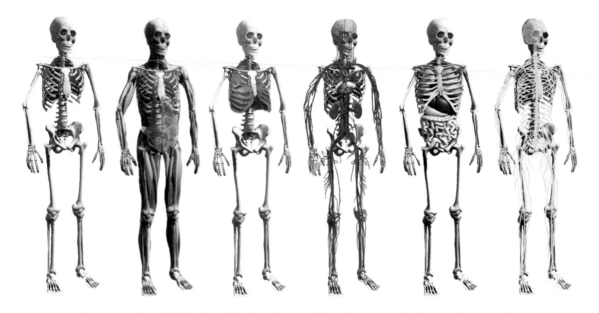

The skeleton as the framework of support for all the body's systems

It makes sense that the many parts of the whole would benefit from maintaining a prescribed orderliness, somewhat like a 3-D puzzle with a place for everything and everything in its place. In an analogy that bears repeating, if the parts of our car's engine were as jumbled as some of our body's organs are, we might have difficulty making it around the block.

Our bodies, while animated by a life force not shared by architectural structures or mechanical engines, still do share a few important features with both of these man-made constructions. Like the engines in our cars, we ingest fuel, convert it to energy, expend the energy, and expel waste products. Our bodily processes are far more complex than this, of course, and require many more detailed steps along

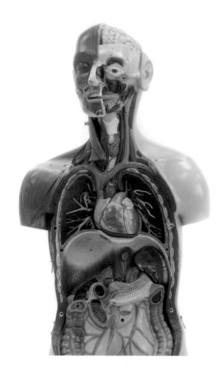

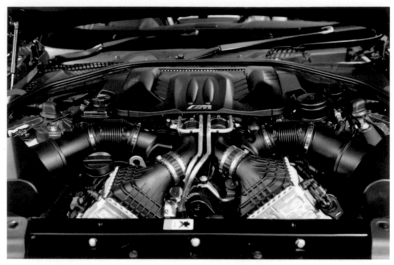

Compare the orderliness of the body's systems with that of a properly functioning car engine. Both must be well maintained in order to function properly.

the way, but the underlying elements remain the same. One has to wonder why, when the efficient operation of a car engine requires that pistons and timing belts be precisely aligned, we give little or no attention to the alignment of the parts in our own personal engine.

ORDERLINESS VS. "DIS-ORDERS"

I am not a doctor or a medically trained health professional. I cannot speak with authority about any of the conditions discussed below. That being said, based on my own experiences and observations and what has been reported to me by others, I have become convinced that structural misalignment plays a far bigger role in many common ailments and conditions than is currently recognized. Evidence of this is only anecdotal at this point. Serious, evidence-based research that examines thriving, healthy—*natural*—models of all ages is calling out to be conducted.

What if cardiovascular disorders were, at least in some cases, related to whether the body is aligned along the vertical axis?

Cardiologists, when consulting with patients who show symptoms of a variety of cardiovascular disorders, will often recommend measures that involve making dietary changes, instituting an exercise regimen, taking prescribed medi-

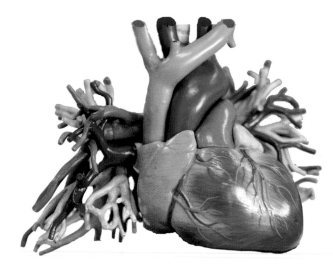

The heart—a three-dimensional organ that relies on open tubes, valves, and chambers to function properly.

cations, and, in some cases, undergoing surgery. This is usually lifesaving advice. It is unlikely, though, that a patient with a chronically collapsed chest or, conversely, a tensely lifted chest is told, "Let's also create space within your chest cavity, front to back and side to side, that keeps the heart, a three-dimensional organ that relies on open tubes, valves, and chambers, from being compressed and distorted."

Blood vessels, which could be compared to miniature garden hoses, also benefit from being unimpeded channels that allow for optimal flow of blood throughout the body. Do we know for sure whether this matters? No, we do not. There appears to be no studies that have looked into this. Ditto for whether the accumulation of plaque in arteries, the accumulation of which is already understood to be related to diet and nutrition, might also have an increased tendency to gather, like silt settling in a pipe, at those places where there is a kink in the hose, so to speak.

The list of symptoms one might experience from cardiovascular problems—pain, shortness of breath, heart palpations, numbness, coughing, weakness, and fatigue—are sometimes treated with expensive medications that can come with potentially serious side effects. "Backward breathing" can cause hyperventilation syndrome, with symptoms that can even mimic a heart attack.[3] People who have learned to realign their bones have often reported great improvement in their ability to breathe more naturally, without stress.

It will be a great day in the world of modern medicine when everyone recognizes how important an aligned body is to overall good health. For this to

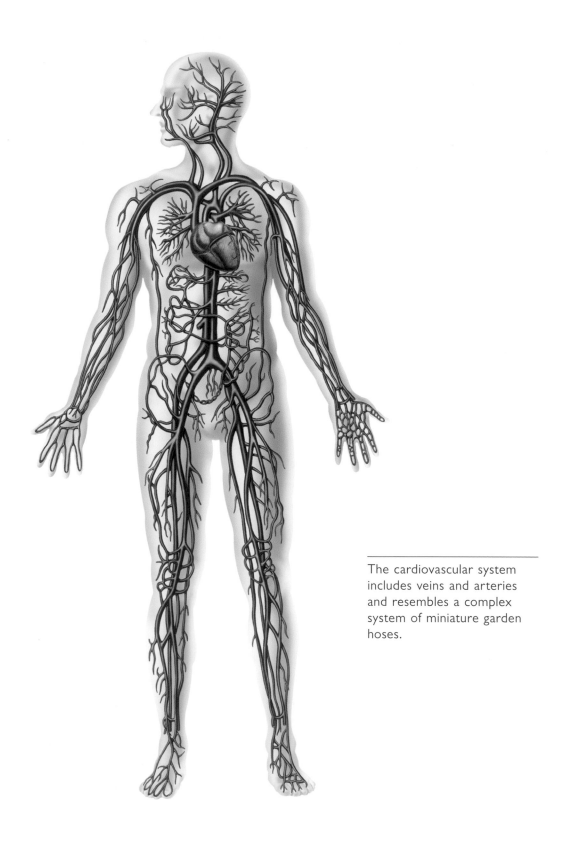

The cardiovascular system includes veins and arteries and resembles a complex system of miniature garden hoses.

happen we must first understand the details of what *naturally healthy* alignment actually is and then include the teaching of this in the standard medical school curriculum.

The body is like a giant symphony orchestra with an almost infinite number of instruments, all of which are interconnected and contribute to the music being produced. None of the body's systems ever plays solo. Each is dependent upon and affected by another. The autonomic nervous system, charged with maintaining a state of equilibrium and homeostasis in all bodily systems and functions, takes its cues from the quality of the breath and tension of the muscles. Likewise, signals from the nervous system trigger a response in the muscles and the respiratory system.

Recommendations for maintaining good health today are focused on three primary factors: diet, exercise, and stress management. Much has been learned and understood about nutrition and which foods support good health and which do not. Much is also understood about the long list of benefits that are to be gained from exercise, although we don't yet recognize the importance of exercising from a natural home base of alignment. As for stress management, many strategies have been developed, most of them based on traditional practices such as meditation, yoga, and breathing and relaxation techniques that help turn down the volume on the high levels of stress that are present in so many people's lives.

A fourth key factor, structural alignment, continues to be overlooked despite its role in providing the underlying framework for the healthy function of all the body's systems. Because the body operates through the interplay of all the parts of each system, this oversight is difficult to understand.

Even today alignment and health have rarely been matched up as a topic for research. For one thing, our culture-wide view of "good posture" does not conform to the body's natural design. The mistaken belief that muscle strength is necessary to hold us up continues to cause many of the joint and pain problems that are treated with therapeutic procedures that often exacerbate the problem, including many surgeries that could be avoided.

Good health equals normal function—no more, no less. Good health, under ordinary conditions, is biologically based and innate to our species—in other words, *natural*. For everyone who is fortunate enough to be born healthy, good health is what we bring into the world and what supports our ability to thrive within a range of normal. Sometimes, if normal is interfered with, even in the name of trying to improve upon it, it is no longer natural.

The most essential ingredients that contribute to good health are clean air and water, a nutritious diet, natural movement, and an ability to relax and renew. While some unavoidable conditions—congenital disorders, certain illnesses, accidents, and natural disasters—are beyond our control, many conditions are within our realm of influence. Lack of clean air or water, a poor diet, lack of healthy movement, and repeated stress all compromise our health. While, tragically, some people have no control over these conditions, many people do.

When we begin to consider just how skeletal alignment might play a role in a number of common health problems and disorders, we begin to see the many ways in which realignment can open many doors to self-healing.

OSTEOARTHRITIS AND HERNIATED DISCS

What if osteoarthritis is largely the result of long-standing habits of unnatural use of the body that have caused repeated compression and wear and tear of joints? Could osteoarthritis be avoided in some cases and improved in others, if people knew how to maintain open space and freedom of movement in their joints through naturally aligning their bones?

Osteoarthritis, which is characterized by inflammation and degeneration of one

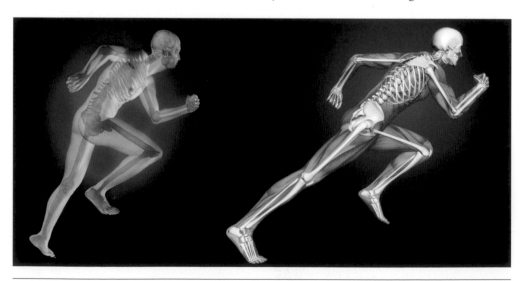

See how the misaligned body places unnatural stress on the joints while running, as compared to the much more efficient aligned body.

or more joints, is the most common reason for disability and joint replacement surgery. Symptoms can be mild to severely painful. Often termed *wear and tear arthritis,* it is commonly believed to be an inevitable consequence of aging for some people and the result of overuse of joints through certain kinds of activities for others.

The kinds of activities in which we participate matter far less than *how* our bodies are aligned when we engage in these activities, whatever they might be. Dysfunctional movement patterns that are not initiated from the deep core put repeated stress on joints, creating imbalance, wearing down cartilage, and restricting range of motion. Learning how to bend in ways that do not stress hips and knees, knowing how to lift and carry a heavy box using the strength of the legs, and understanding how to swing a golf club or a tennis racket so that the shoulders do not strain are all ways that osteoarthritis can be avoided by relieving compression in our joints. Most important, having a strong core facilitates a natural traction of the spine and a lifting of weight and compression off the body's joints. In those cases where there has not yet been serious degradation of cartilage, applying these measures can often bring relief from, and even reverse, stiffness and pain.

What if a herniated disc is the result of chronic misalignment that causes compression of certain segments within the cervical, thoracic, or lumbar spine? People with a strong core, that naturally keeps the spine elongated, are not likely to suffer the terrible pain of a herniated, or bulging, disc. This injury can be a long time in the making or can occur quite suddenly when turning to the side or lifting something heavy. Either way, except for accidents that occasionally occur, a herniated disc is almost always the result of the kind of compression that results from misalignment in the spine.

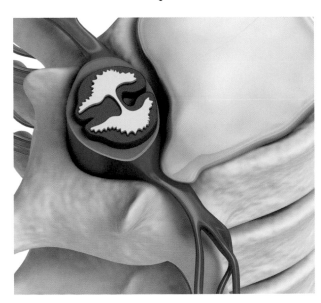

A herniated disc is one in which pressure on an intervertebral disc pushes the disc beyond its natural boundaries, impinging on a nerve.

The terminology describing a herniated disc can be confusing because many different terms—herniated disc, slipped disc, bulging disc, degenerative disc disease—are sometimes used interchangeably so that a precise assessment is not always clear.

In the most extreme cases the disc may be said to be ruptured, wherein the nucleus is squeezed beyond the wall of the disc and leaks into the spinal canal. This can be caused by traumatic injury but is far more commonly caused by habits of use that put continuous pressure on one or more discs through chronic collapse of the structure of the spine. Something as minor as bending to the side to pick up something can trigger a major episode.

Not all herniated discs cause pain and some, even the ones that are painful, appear to repair themselves on occasion. Studies reveal that the spine lengthens in some people during the course of a night's sleep, presumably due to an increase in the water content of the disc when the spine, which was compressed during the day like a sponge being squeezed, is plumped up again while lying down. Squeezed dry, the disc flattens and becomes brittle. Eventually it crumbles and falls apart and is said to be a desiccated disc. When a constantly squeezed disc deteriorates to the point where it can no longer rehydrate, the facets between the vertebrae rub against each other, resulting in ongoing pain.

Learning how to naturally extend the spine by turning on the power button at the core while sitting, standing, and engaging in everyday activities is the most effective way to address this problem in the long term, both in terms of prevention and treatment.

OSTEOPOROSIS

What if the development of osteoporosis were influenced by one's lifelong postural habits, contributing to the creation of certain conditions that might make some people more susceptible to a process of gradual bone loss than others?

Osteoporosis is a common condition characterized by a high level of bone loss, putting people at increased risk of fractures and general spinal deterioration. The progression of the bone loss often goes undiagnosed unless one has a bone density test or suffers a fracture. The risk of hip and spinal fractures is especially high in the older population, among whom osteoporosis is particularly common. As the disease progresses a succession of vertebral fractures, sometimes indiscernible at the time, can lead to a gradual collapse of the spine and has been described as resulting in noticeable rounding of the upper back.

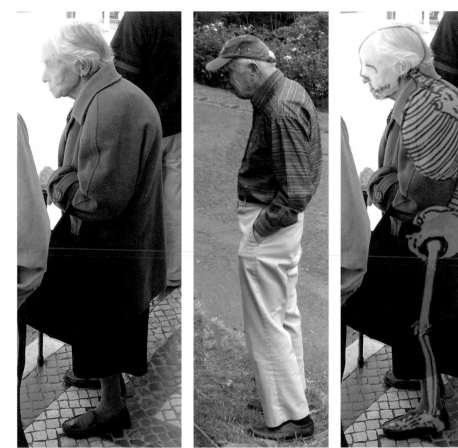
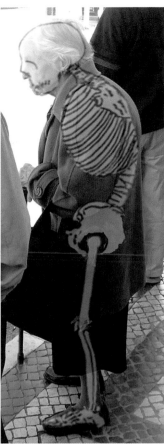
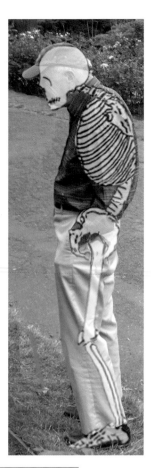

These people likely spent many years with misaligned posture, resulting in the spinal deterioration you now see.

Until recently, loss of bone density was considered the primary cause of spinal collapse in the elderly, but new evidence has been coming to light revealing that not everyone who displays a severely rounded spine (what has been termed *advanced, observable osteoporosis*) has significant bone loss.[4] The surprising discovery that kyphosis (the often-referred-to dowager's hump) may not be the outcome of poor bone density, points now to lifelong skeletal misalignment as playing a significant role in structural collapse.

Bone loss is a serious health problem because of the high risk of bone fractures that can result from it. What may have gone unnoticed in the current research is that fractures may be far more likely to occur (barring traumatic falls) when the body is misaligned to begin with. Such misalignment causes unnatural movement patterns, such as bending forward with a curved or arched spine. People who bend as they did as babies, by hinging at the hips and maintaining the natural elongation of the spine, do not put undue pressure on the vertebrae. Many spinal fractures occur when the spine is compressed while something is being lifted or the torso is twisting to the side. The posture one has had over many years may play a far more significant role in the incidence of nontraumatic bone fractures than has been recognized and may explain why more than half of the people with existing osteoporosis never experience a fracture, while many others, with normal bone density, do fracture bones.

A search of the medical literature turns up this list of the most commonly accepted causes of osteoporosis:

- an inherited predisposition,
- low calcium intake,
- insufficient vitamin D,
- poor calcium absorption,
- lack of sufficient weight-bearing activity,
- lack of exercise, and
- change in reproductive hormones.

While any or all of these factors may play an important part, it is remarkable that no mention is made that skeletal alignment or postural habits might play a role in any way whatsoever. Considering the problems caused by this condition for millions of people, this appears to be a stunning oversight.

Medical treatment methods for osteoporosis usually involve the taking of bisphosphonates, a class of drugs that has been shown to improve bone density in many instances but which can also cause serious side effects. New evidence has come to light recently that vitamin D, in adequate doses, is more important for the absorption of calcium than previously recognized. An alkaline, plant-based diet is important for avoiding bone loss as well as rebuilding bone, whereas a diet with an acidic pH contributes to further bone loss. Exercise, such as walking that is done briskly and with weight borne solidly through a deeply connected heel, also shows evidence of contributing to bone health. As usual, skeletal alignment and *how* weight is borne through the entire skeleton is rarely mentioned, even in connection with weight-bearing exercises. Too often natural alignment is either overlooked completely, or, in those rare instances when alignment is mentioned, true natural alignment continues to be misunderstood.

Given that anecdotal evidence points to almost everyone who has advanced observable osteoporosis as having had a retroverted pelvis for many years, it is clear that research must examine the relationship between osteoporosis and bone fractures and a spine that has not had the support of a well-anchored pelvis.

As with almost every other area affecting overall health, there is a lack of research that takes the body's natural alignment into consideration. This is especially important in the face of an overreliance on drugs now coming under increased scrutiny for serious side effects, including, ironically, spontaneous bone fractures.[5] Research that examines the postural habits of people who develop osteoporosis could also lead to understanding how other possible causes of this disease might interrelate with each other.

While some research has been conducted that compares the incidence of osteoporosis among different cultures in the world, the emphasis of these studies has primarily been on diet and lifestyle and has not included differences that relate to the alignment of the skeleton. Studies that track the bone density and postural habits of people diagnosed with osteopenia (early-stage bone loss) could reveal whether adopting improved postural alignment could help to reverse the progression of bone loss.

THE RELATION OF SKELETAL ALIGNMENT TO SPINAL DISORDERS

What if skeletal alignment plays a role in contributing to the development of many of the most commonly diagnosed disorders of the spine such as kyphosis, lordosis, sciatica, spinal stenosis, spondylolisthesis, and degenerative disc disease?

Millions of people receive the diagnosis of one or more of these complicated and somewhat frightening-sounding conditions while often being left to believe that little can be done to help these problems other than managing their pain. While other factors are involved in some instances, the great majority of back pain problems are the result of structural misalignment and dysfunctional movement patterns. I know this to be true by the number of people I have seen reverse, or at least greatly improve, a number of these conditions. It is uncanny how often people who have "tried everything," even surgery in some instances, have found the wherewithal *within themselves,* to find relief from long-standing conditions, no matter their age.

The majority of spinal conditions are caused, barring accidents, by a particular structural imbalance that, when chronic over a number of years, leads to their development. The more we understand the details of these conditions, the more we will be able to guide our own process in remediating our posture to avoid or relieve them. The chart below will be of assistance in relating the misaligned stances we have discussed to the conditions that can result from them.

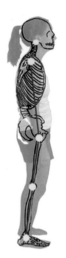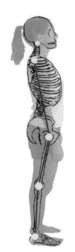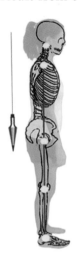

Spinal Conditions and the Stances That Cause Them

Condition Name	Description	Stance at Fault (In Figure above)
Kyphosis	Excessive rounding of the thoracic spine (upper back)	Left
Lordosis	Excessive arching of the lumbar spine (lower back), often referred to as swayback	Middle
Sciatica	Pain, weakness, tingling, or numbness in the lower back, buttocks, or legs due to pressure on the sciatic nerve in the lower spine	Left or middle depending upon where the pressure occurs
Spondylosis	Degenerative osteoarthritis of certain joints of the spine	Left or middle depending where the distortion and impingement occur
L5 spondylolisthesis	Forward slippage of one vertebra relative to the one beneath it	Middle
Degenerative disc disease	Deterioration of one or more intervertebral discs of the spine, this diagnosis is not necessarily degenerative, nor is it a disease	Left or middle depending where the deterioration and compression occur
Spinal stenosis	Narrowing of the spinal column or openings where spinal nerves leave the spinal column	Left or middle depending where the narrowing occurs

The structurally aligned figure on the right is unlikely to develop any of these conditions, even if she were to engage in heavy labor and carry heavy things on her head. The position of her pelvis supports a spine that is not distorted or compressed. Her core is automatically engaged in almost everything that she does, not only stabilizing her spine but also elongating it so that compression and nerve impingement are never a factor. Her joints are loose, yet stable, able to move with ease and free of any stiffness.

BREATHING AND STRESS

What if skeletal alignment plays a role in certain respiratory disorders influenced by whether diaphragmatic muscle fibers are askew or in a natural configuration?

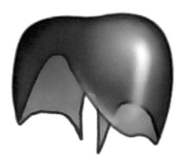

The diaphragm, as the primary muscle of respiration, requires that the rib cage to which it attaches is in a naturally aligned position so that it can contract and relax naturally with each breath.

TRY IT ON!

The Diaphragm and Easeful Breathing

When you breathe from the support of an aligned skeleton, the breath rises and falls from deep within, softly filling the back and the sides of the torso as well as the front. The following exercise will give you a sense of how movement of the diaphragm is restricted by misalignment.

- Let yourself completely collapse into a slouched heap. (Only do this if this does not cause you to feel pain anywhere.)
- Notice that your pelvis is tucked into a sad dog position and your back is rounded and collapsed. Feel your rib cage sinking into your abdomen.
- Chances are your chin is out in front of you and the back of your neck is compressed. Let's hope you don't really sit this slouched, but this is what it feels like for the millions of people who do.

- Draw in three slow, deep breaths and notice how this feels.
- Are you able to sense the movement of your diaphragm? Where in your torso do you feel your breath?
- Now lift your chest as high as you can, and pull your shoulders way back. (Again, only do this if this does not cause you to feel pain anywhere.)
- Do you notice your back arching? What about tension in your neck or anywhere else?
- Notice the position of your head and chin. Is your neck relaxed?
- Draw in three slow, deep breaths and notice how this feels.
- Are you able to sense the movement of your diaphragm? Where in your torso do you feel your breath?
- Now reestablish a happy dog pelvis. On the next exhalation, relax your chest downward, feeling your back growing wide. Do not worry about your shoulders for this exercise. Let your chin drop slightly so that the back of the neck is comfortably long and soft.
- Now draw in three slow, deep breaths and notice how this feels.
- Are you able to sense the movement of your diaphragm? Where in your torso do you feel your breath? Do you feel it filling the torso more completely in every direction?

Collapsing the chest or artificially lifting it upward are unnatural conditions that distort the fibers of the diaphragm and disrupt its ability to gently rise and fall with each relaxed breath. In extreme cases distortion of the diaphragm and thoracic cavity can contribute to such stress-related disorders as chronic hyperventilation syndrome, anxiety, and panic attacks. It is not uncommon for these stress conditions to mimic symptoms of chest pain and heart attack that sometimes clear up quickly when natural, relaxed breathing is restored.

Stress kills. One way it does this is by triggering sympathetic nervous system dominance that interferes with the immune system's ability to ward off infections and diseases. From a purely scientific perspective, skeletal alignment is not yet recognized as playing any role in promoting stress, but it is hard to imagine this won't change when the body's natural alignment is finally recognized as essential to the healthy functioning of all the body's systems and a key component to good overall health.

Because researchers limit their observations to third person subjects and do not become the subjects of their own experiments, certain details that can only be discovered through direct experience are slow to rise to the surface as points worthy of scientific study. Nevertheless, just about anyone can experience the tension that gathers along the length of the spine by tucking the tailbone, sucking in the belly, lifting the chest, lifting the chin, and holding this for a minute or two.

This is the stance of "Attention" in the military command, juxtaposed with the relief that is experienced at the sound of the words "At Ease." Ironically, many people take this same overlifted stance when practicing *tadasana,* or Mountain pose, in yoga, misunderstanding the intention of the pose in representing a mountain that is solid and serenely present rather than a giant rumbling mound of tension. Aligning the bones doesn't get rid of the basic stresses of daily life, but it can go far in creating the conditions that make it possible to navigate these stresses with much greater ease.

Among other diseases and disorders that can be made worse, or in some cases even caused by skeletal misalignment, is acid reflux disorder. Physical displacement,

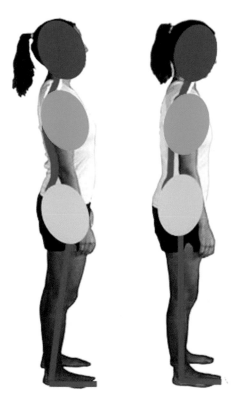

The tension in the back that accompanies lifting the chest (rib cage wheel rolling backward) affects the sympathetic nervous system (fright, fight-or-flight) and is often experienced in the body as a chronic, low-level state of alarm.

impingement, or distortion of the small valve at the entrance of the stomach, the lower esophageal sphincter, most likely plays a significant role in acid reflux or GERD (gastroesophageal reflux disorder). Medical texts describe this condition as being caused by the valve not functioning properly, a weakness in the diaphragm, or a stomach abnormality. More specifically, a hiatal hernia, a bulge where a part of the stomach protrudes at the opening where the esophagus normally passes through the diaphragm, is frequently blamed.

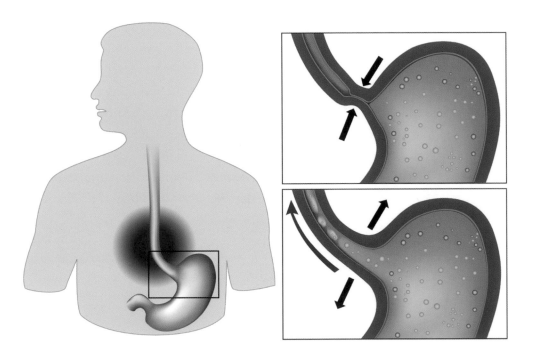

The pinching of the valve at the entrance to the stomach causing gastric reflux

Remarkably, the cause of a hiatal hernia is almost always said to be unknown, although it is unlikely it just happens in a vacuum, for no reason. Postural collapse, which most surely can cause impingement of the esophageal valve, is never considered, in spite of the fact that an uncountable number of people struggle with this condition and typically treat it with a variety of medications. It also comes as no surprise that the sudden rise of this condition among children today coincides with the growing collapse of their framework of support.

KEEPING AN OPEN FLOW TO THE BRAIN

The brain and its many complex functions require a constant supply of oxygen that is delivered in the form of oxygenated blood, pumped through the neck and head by the carotid and vertebral arteries. When blood flow is cut off to the brain (*ischemia*), healthy brain function diminishes rapidly. A study of the literature related to cerebral blood flow reveals that it is determined by several factors: the viscosity of the blood, how dilated blood vessels are, and the net pressure of the flow of blood into the brain.

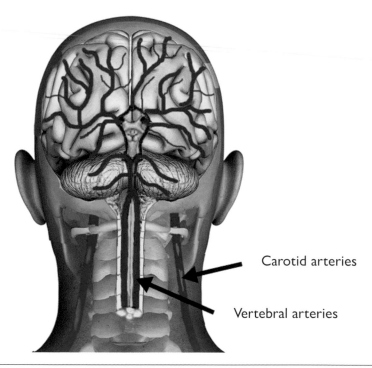

Carotid arteries

Vertebral arteries

The carotid arteries (along the front and side of the neck) and the vertebral arteries (along the spine) supply blood to the neck, head, face, and brain, distributing nourishing oxygen to billions of neurons.

Cerebral blood vessels are able to change the flow of blood through autoregulation, constricting and dilating the diameter of the blood vessels to adjust to changing levels of blood pressure. The vertebral arteries, as well as branches of the basilar artery that penetrates the brainstem, are especially common sites of occlusion, the narrowing or cutting off of blood flowing to the brain.

This would help explain why a small number of older women have experienced "beauty parlor syndrome," an ischemic attack or stroke that occurs while having their hair washed at a beauty parlor.[6] Though rare, this particular stroke appears to be caused by the sharp angle of the neck when the head is tipped back, cutting off the flow of blood through the vertebral arteries or overstretching and tearing the carotid artery in the front of the neck.

Strokes are usually caused by blockage of the flow of blood in one of the arteries to the brain. High risk factors are high cholesterol, high blood pressure, obesity, diabetes, and other factors related to cardiovascular issues brought about through smoking, poor nutrition, and a sedentary lifestyle. Clearly this accounts in large part for the sudden climb in the number of strokes among children and young adults that has risen as overall health has declined. Between 1994 and 2007 there was an increase of more than 30 percent in children five to fourteen years old, and this figure was even higher in the fifteen- to thirty-four-year age group.[7]

Without maximum, efficient blood flow to the brain, students might find it difficult to focus and concentrate, at best.

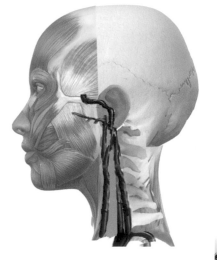
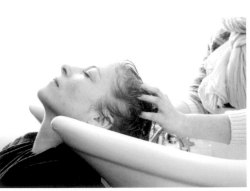
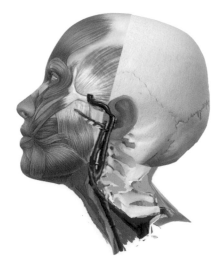

These images show how the arteries can be compromised when the head is tilted back, resulting in beauty parlor syndrome. It seems likely that those women who are most susceptible to this occurring are those who have had a history of compression in the neck.

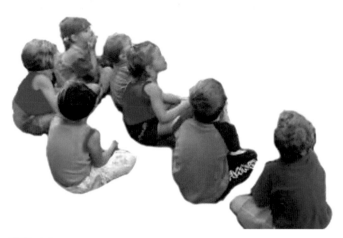

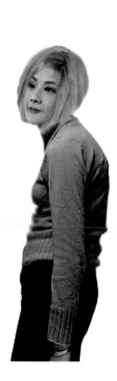

Is it far-fetched to suggest that some children and young adults, like those pictured here, are continuously reinforcing a "beauty parlor neck" and adversely affecting blood flow to the brain and all other organs of the body? The head is quite heavy, after all, being similar in weight to a bowling ball. Dropping it backward and continuously pressing it down on life-sustaining arteries and the spinal cord may result in serious consequences.

10

BEYOND THE PHYSICAL

AS WE LEARN HOW to apply principles of natural alignment into our daily activities, it becomes readily apparent that, in order for us to be successful with this, we have to pay close attention to our present-moment experience. To apply mindfulness to our physical alignment we must invite a recurring and gradual process that directs awareness inside our skin, again and again, to include the physical body as well as the thinking, perceiving mind.

Mindfulness is the experience of moment-by-moment awareness. It can be cultivated through a formal practice of meditation, often based on traditional Eastern practices, or it can be built and strengthened by anchoring our focus on the body as the object of our awareness as we move through the tasks of daily living. Mindfulness provides us with options for how to navigate our automatic, conditioned responses and helps us learn to recognize what is happening in *this* moment. By cultivating mindfulness we have an opportunity to observe ourselves and to choose how we might respond, if at all, to our experience. Being present with ourselves in this way is strictly a solo endeavor that no one else can do for us or to us. In the end, it is up to each one of us, and only if we choose, to discover what it means to be a wholly awakened and enlivened body and mind. Life goes on, whether or not we are mindful, but the choice to be more mindful can enrich our lives in uncountable ways.

HOW MEDITATION CAN HELP

Mindfulness meditation, as a formal practice, is designed to train the mind to be more aware. We may have been continuously aware of our experience as babies and

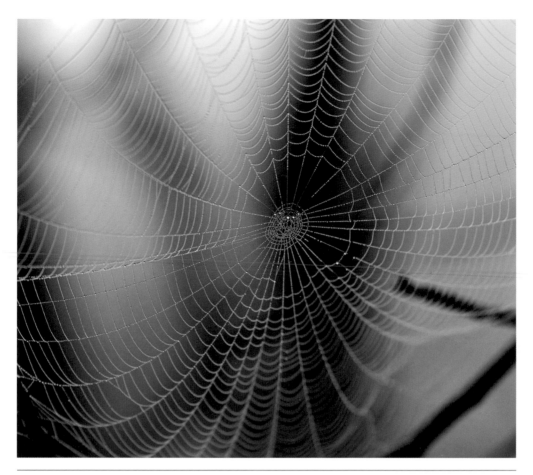

We must be as aware of our physical alignment as the spider is of its intricately woven web.

very young children, but for most of us such awareness has been trumped by the development of an overly active thinking mind. Whenever we make an effort to maintain awareness of something as simple as the rising and falling of the breath or the subtle sensations of the body, we soon realize how quickly our attention has traveled elsewhere. We might try again, still without success, believing now that our mind is just too active for mediation. This is why many people give up right at the beginning.

If we do not give up, but instead keep returning to the breath again and again—and *again*—we may experience glimpses of quietude that are compelling enough to draw us in further. We become curious and interested in knowing what happens if we continue.

Mindfulness meditation has proven to be so effective in reducing stress and improving overall health that it has been successfully incorporated into hundreds of hospital programs around the United States. New developments in neuroscience and magnetic resonance imaging (MRI) reveal that the brain shows significant gray matter density growth in areas of the brain involved in learning, memory, empathy, compassion, and emotional regulation in people who meditated for as little as eight weeks, as compared to a control group.[1] In addition, the researchers referred to an earlier study that found a correlation between decreased gray matter in the *amygdala,* a region of the brain that affects fear and stress, and a reduction in self-reported stress levels. Meditation helps to improve a number of health complaints, such as high blood pressure, anxiety, depression, chronic pain, and insomnia, as well as boosting the immune system.[2]

One easily understood way that mindfulness meditation appears to work is in turning down the volume on the sympathetic (fight-or-flight, stress) aspect of the nervous system, that part of the nervous system that drives emotional states such as fear, anger, and frustration and can be the culprit in insomnia and panic attacks. Reducing sympathetic nervous system involvement allows the parasympathetic nervous system to play a more balancing, calming role.

So what could alignment of one's bones possibly have to do with affecting things such as gray matter density and decreases in stress? Natural alignment is a bonus to meditators in several important ways.

Those people who struggle with physical pain while meditating can greatly lessen, and often completely eliminate, *unnecessary* pain. *How* we sit while meditating is key to what our experience will be. Some people practice meditation for many years and continue to encounter recurring pain that is caused by a lack of support of aligned bones. While some pain will always be a part of meditation practice, much unnecessary pain is endured through a belief that we must transcend the body rather than understand and live by its natural design. Some longtime meditators develop serious, debilitating physical problems from years of practicing with a compressed spine and restricted joints. It doesn't have to be this way. Aligned bones provide the framework of support for much of the freedom that can be gained in the body and mind through meditation.

Aligned bones, and the conscious awareness of them, can serve as a solid, concrete anchor to the present that draws the witnessing mind bone deep, to the very marrow of our physical existence. Awareness of our bones, like our breath, is forever available to us, and knowing how they relate to each other for greatest freedom from tension can help to sharpen our concentration.

Finally, aligned bones support the flow of energy, blood, lymph, interstitial fluids, and a continuous stream of consciousness that can be blocked by the mistaken notion that the mind and body are separate. This is yet another way we try to transcend the body, when inhabiting it fully is what puts it at peace with itself and in harmony with the world around it.

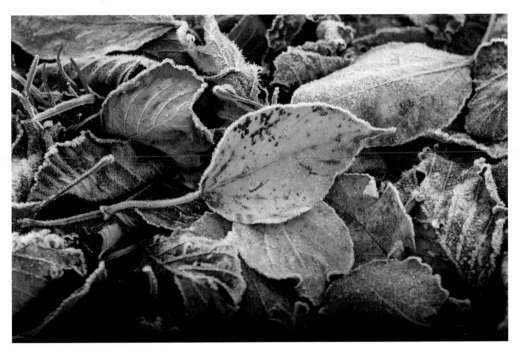

The healthy body is no more separate from the mind than a healthy leaf is separate from the tree. As the leaf begins to wither and die when it is separated from the tree, so the mind lacks harmony when it is disconnected from the aligned body. It is only when they are fully connected that they are both in harmony.

Meditation is never easy for anyone. Encounters with physical and emotional pain will always be a part of the process. Included in meditation instructions are helpful, liberating techniques for using pain to navigate the five hindrances—negative mind states described in Buddhist teaching that can stymie the practice and stand in the way of happiness and contentment. These hindrances are *attachment* (to that which we want), *aversion* (to that which we don't want), *restlessness* (agitations of the mind and body), *laziness* (drowsiness and mental torpor), and *doubt* (lack of fortitude and trust in the benefits of the process). It is only partially in jest that the suggestion is made here that if the historical Buddha were to walk among us today he might include a sixth hindrance: unnatural posture. While not a mental state, as are the others, structural misalignment and lack of a strong core of internal support contribute to feeding all the other hindrances. The Buddha, in spite of his wisdom, would not have had to consider this back at a time when most people were likely to inhabit their bodies in a naturally aligned way.

As we develop greater skill at being mindful, we gradually become more adept at noticing how we are sitting, getting out of a chair, reaching to a high shelf, opening a door, driving a car, running a race, bending to tie a shoe, or lifting a child. We become more practiced at being our natural, pain-free, mindful self, where almost continuous mindfulness of the body becomes an anchor to our present experience, whatever we are doing. In this way we are meditating all day long.

Choosing to be mindful in regular daily living is not an easy thing to do. Focusing on our presently occurring experience means we will sometimes encounter physical, mental, and emotional conditions that we would rather avoid. It's quite natural that we might prefer to hide out from feeling painful emotions or sensations in the body. Almost everyone's tendency is to want to avoid just about anything that makes us uncomfortable. We want joy, not sadness; security, not fear; pleasure, not pain. Peace dwells at a place of equanimity in the middle and comes from an acceptance of what is.

Most of us will read a book, watch TV, go to a movie, work overtime, call a friend, read the news, go to the gym, drink a beer, eat a snack, go shopping, surf the net, take a nap, watch more TV, have another snack—all common, normal everyday activities that are not inherently bad or wrong and that anyone can feel free to enjoy. The problem arises when we relentlessly stack one mindless activity on top of another—and yet another—until we have limited our ability to tune in with awareness to what is really going on, emotionally and physically, underneath all the business. We don't notice, perhaps, that some of our strategies for avoiding mental tension or physical discomfort are at the root of what might be causing that issue in the first place.

Simply avoiding what is unpleasant, whether it is physical or mental, often leads to more of the same down the road. This is especially true if the cause of the pain is overlooked and the symptoms are covered up or masked. Taking pain medication for chronic back pain that could otherwise be resolved (if we or our doctors only knew how) is an example of one very common way of avoiding pain that still lurks under the surface. Pain is a signal, a call to attention. One of the most effective ways to address the problem of pain and discomfort, by either alleviating or learning to manage it, is to develop greater awareness through a practice of mindfulness.

Mindfulness, by cultivating awareness of our present experience in an ongoing process of investigation and discovery, without judgment, gives us tools to cope with what seems unacceptable or even unbearable. Simply deciding to be mindful is not enough, though, as anyone who takes up this practice soon learns. Mindfulness can only be contacted in each moment, and in the beginning, more often than not, it is lost in the next. Soon, however, mindful moments grow in number and become strung together. We experience stretches of "the one moment," that is always *this* moment, and we recognize the ways in which our lives are enhanced by this awakening to presence.

OPENING CHANNELS

The concept of energy moving in the body has been a focal point of spiritual traditions and practices for thousands of years and plays a significant role in martial arts, yoga, Chinese medicine, and other approaches to spirituality and health that have become popular in the West today. Chakras, described as "vortices of bioenergetic activity emanating from the major nerve ganglia branching forward from the spinal column," have their origin in ancient Hindu texts.[3] Purported to be centers of consciousness within the subtle body, chakras cannot be touched or seen when autopsies are conducted, so they are often dismissed as being imaginary and having no basis in physical fact. Even so, mountains of recorded information from a variety of traditions have described chakras in great detail as they relate to experiences of expanded consciousness.

Whether the primary chakras are aligned is said to greatly affect physical health, a sense of place in the world, emotional well-being, and relationships with others. Some people employ a variety of methods to align their chakras, including visualization exercises, meditation, dietary measures, acupuncture, and physical exercises. Ironically, even though the chakras are located along the central energy channel, or *sushumna nadi,* which corresponds with the physical spine and central nervous system, natural alignment of the skeleton itself is rarely mentioned in terms of what role, if any, it might play in aligned chakras. This further demonstrates a common disconnection that exists in our culture that sets body and spirit apart, as if not interrelated but separate from one another, as if science and the sacred could be anything other than one and the same, or as if the earth and humans or any other living thing are not just pieces of one great integrated whole.

When we examine physical details that relate to spiritual practices we begin to

Opening our hearts and letting down our guard in this way can be a scary proposition, because removing the shield leaves us vulnerable to many things—to being hurt, to letting others in, to feeling the pain against which we've worked so hard to protect ourselves, sometimes since a long-ago childhood. Yet this willingness to be vulnerable is the hallmark of an open heart. It requires an ability to trust in the face of fear, to feel safe in the middle of uncertainty, and to find strength within ourselves when we are feeling weak and insecure. Finding the natural, *physical* support that exists within us as an unfailing architectural underpinning empowers us with a bone deep strength all our own that helps us to feel safe enough to trust, even in difficult times.

BODY AS METAPHOR

Psychological and emotional states are often reflected in the way we inhabit the body, as evidenced by many of the expressions we use to describe people. The words *he is full of himself* are likely to conjure up an image of someone with a puffed-up chest and whose energetic presence is directed into the front of the body (head and rib cage wheels rolled backward). This is a different image from the one seen by the mind's eye when hearing someone described as being spineless, having no backbone, or being weak-kneed (rib cage wheel forward and pelvic wheel back). One can be a pain in the neck because one keeps a stiff upper lip, has feet of clay, is an anal-retentive tight-ass (pelvic wheel rolled backward), and turns a deaf ear. This is not the same as having your head in the clouds and, therefore, not having a leg to stand on. These are not just random expressions that landed in our language without meaning but windows that may sometimes offer a glimpse into psychological and emotional aspects of our psychological being.

Chances are you look quite different when you are feeling depressed and low than you do when you are feeling excited and up. Then again, there is the middle way of equanimity—neither up nor down, but centered—where the bones are aligned and the energy is calm. This fundamental energy is the ground of our being; the stream of consciousness that is either flowing freely at any given moment or getting bogged down. Skeletal alignment sets up the physical conditions necessary for facilitating our ability to fully participate in this flow.

Accomplished actors use subtle details of skeletal alignment, whether or not they know it, in creating the characters who temporarily inhabit their bodies. An actor can draw upon many traits when playing the part of someone who is stuck up, looks down the nose at people, is arrogant, and has a condescending attitude. This actor is likely to lift the chin skyward (a requirement for looking down the nose), pin the shoulders back, and hold the chest up with mountains of tension.

It's important that we not overdo sweeping generalizations as they relate to a complex issue that is, in actuality, beyond the scope of our understanding. Obviously many factors are involved in contributing to the totality of our physical and emotional being, some of which are beyond our conscious control. Not everyone who has a perpetually lifted chin has a condescending attitude any more than a person who has perfect natural posture is friendly and kind. However, everyone with a lifted-up chin *does* have compression in the cervical spine, along with whatever kinds of resulting constriction, blockage, and tension may (or may not) contribute to a particular attitude. Curiously, the word *attitude,* while meaning "to have a particular perspective on something," also means "taking a certain physical posture, especially while interacting with others." Over and over again we find cues in our language that point to the likelihood that the connections between the physical, psychological, and spiritual aspects of being may have been understood long ago. It may be only in recent history that we have become disconnected enough from our center to have lost sight of certain understandings we once had.

Off-center skeletons are not aligned with the present. An actor portraying someone stuck in the past, filled with regret, whose mantra is "if only," would slouch and sink, behind the axis, as if the body itself could be collapsed into the past. What posture would you take if you were striving to get ahead, checking things off a mile-long to-do list? An actor playing the role of this type A personality would be lifting the chest and leaning forward of the axis.

This is, of course, an oversimplification, but there is more than a smattering of truth in these physical stereotypes. How would the bones be organized in a body that reflected shyness? A sense of entitlement? Overwhelming grief? For some people these mental states can become a chronic condition, along with the aches and pains and stiff joints that are part and parcel of these postures.

As a young mother I was plagued with recurring back pain that frequently sent me to a chiropractor, an almost constantly aching hip that kept me awake some nights, chronically tight shoulders, and headaches and other symptoms of TMJ (temporomandibular joint disorder). Massages brought relief, but only for a short time. In my late twenties I took up aerobic exercises, and sometime after that I was introduced to yoga by a visiting friend who agreed to give classes in my falling short, is the closest expression found in English that describes a center of knowing at the core. This is another example of how expressions we sometimes use without understanding their origins can tell us what our ancestors might have known that we have long since forgotten.

Throughout the ages, artists have created paintings and statues of well-known spiritual icons such as Jesus and the Buddha. While these artists may not have been naturally aligned themselves, they nevertheless seem to have intuited what the posture of peacefulness looks like. Such representations of peace almost always reflect qualities of alignment, symmetry, and balance. These are frequently seen in nature and man-made structures, all of which are governed by natural, scientific laws.

Other qualities may be evident in artists' renditions as well, but these are *sensed* by the observer more than they can be easily described, such as a solid strength that is neither rigid nor hard, a gentleness that is not weak or collapsed, a calm equanimity that is not disengaged. How is it that such amorphous qualities

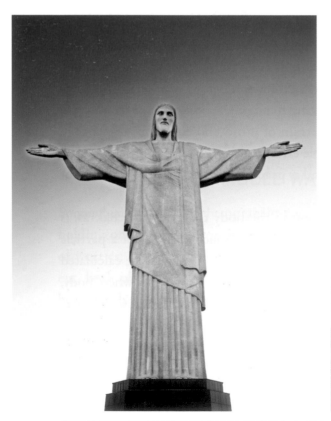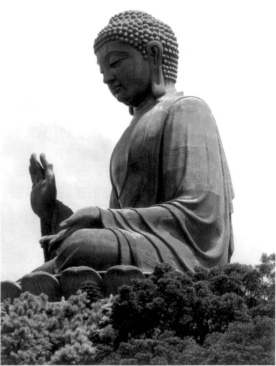

Notice how these statues embody an inherently natural alignment.

seem to emanate from within an inanimate painting or stone statue? What is the essence within the gracefully draping folds of a monk's robes that awakens a sense of reverence in so many people when they view these images?

Natural alignment describes that place where we align with our own nature, a place we recognize as being familiar, a coming home to what is inborn and unchanging. In the mixture of power and grace we see in a statue of Jesus or the Buddha, we may see a reflection of ourselves that harkens back to moments in time when we have known how to trust and feel safe. We too are powerful yet yielding; solid to the core, yet soft and permeable. These are not opposites that tear us apart but different sides of a coin that can be balanced on its edge—the middle way. Dwelling in the mysterious unknown does not have to be experienced as a threat so much as an adventure that can be enjoyed through a ground of acceptance and trust that comes with aligning ourselves with all aspects of our whole, integrated self. In specifically physical terms this ground is provided by a core of well-being made possible by the underlying framework of an aligned skeleton and elastic muscles.

BALANCE IN THE BELLY

Gut feelings can be difficult to consciously experience when they are locked inside rock-hard "killer abs" or a core that is deadened by collapse. We live in a culture that reveres abdominal muscles that can be seen on the surface of the body. Even mannequins modeling bathing suits in store windows are now being manufactured to proudly display flat, rippling sections of muscle. Many health-related magazines will have at least one article per issue on how to flatten your belly in ten days or less. Unfortunately many of the exercises designed to do this only entrench tension patterns that repeatedly compress the spine and tighten the diaphragm, thus restricting natural, relaxed breathing. As a culture that is focused on working out at the gym we are binding ourselves up with more and more tension while our greatest freedom lies in the boundless peace available to us when those tensions are released. Our muscle-obsessed culture (strengthen them, stretch them) must now look deeper, to the bones that first must be aligned, in order to let our straining muscles off the hook.

Genuine strength and power originate in a belly that is open to experiencing life as it moves through us. The act of breathing delivers oxygen from outside the body into the lungs, where it is then pumped as oxygenated blood throughout the

It is a curious fact that the root of the word *sacrum,* on which the spine sits, is the same as the Latin root for the word *sacred.* The Greek words for sacrum, *hieron osteon,* mean "holy bone," indicating that this bone has long been considered as having particular significance. Made up of five fused vertebrae, the sacrum is a plug that fits between the two sides of the pelvis and provides a platform for the spine. In the yogic tradition the spine is considered to be the seat of consciousness. In this context the sacrum then becomes the "seat of the seat" of consciousness and the ground from which the sleeping *kundalini* or *shakti* energy awakens.

Artists who depict the various prophets and deities of the world show us, beyond words, that peace is an "inside job," a continuous flow of life that is free of all tensions of mind and body, made possible when we are aligned with the most basic laws of nature.

Peace, it seems, has the potential to be an equally universal and profoundly personal experience that always "begins with me."

PART TWO

■ ■ ■

Putting It All Together

Think with the whole body.
Taisen Deshimaru

HOW TO SIT

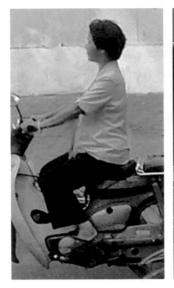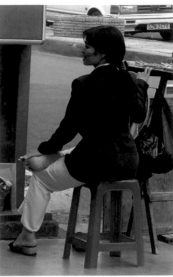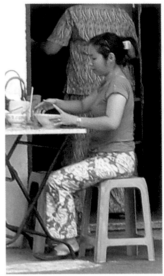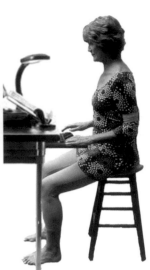

Sitting in an aligned position is critical to true health and fitness.

- Establish your solid seat on an anchored pelvis. You may want to sit on a wedge-shaped cushion. (See resources.)
- Relax the belly.
- Release the front of your chest downward as your back rises up behind you. As your back rises, your core will engage (power button).
- Roll one shoulder, then the other, onto the top of the rib cage (fasten the shoulders).
- Drop your chin slightly. Sense the front of the throat sliding (without tension) toward the back of the throat, then floating upward. The back of the neck lengthens (neck sweep).
- Look straight ahead by using your eyes, not your head, to look up.
- Observe the gentle rising and falling away of the breath.

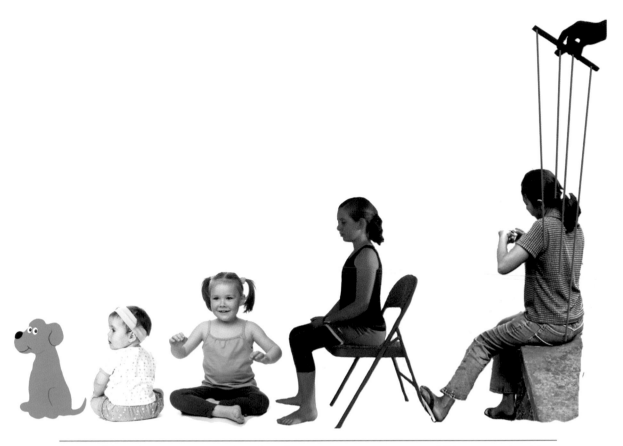

As we did without conscious thought when we were very young children, we should now be mindful of our alignment and maintain a happy dog stance.

Sitting Shortcut

- Sit on your sitz bones.
- Relax your belly.
- Release your chest down.
- Fasten your shoulders.
- Do a neck sweep.
- Let your bones support you.

HOW TO STAND

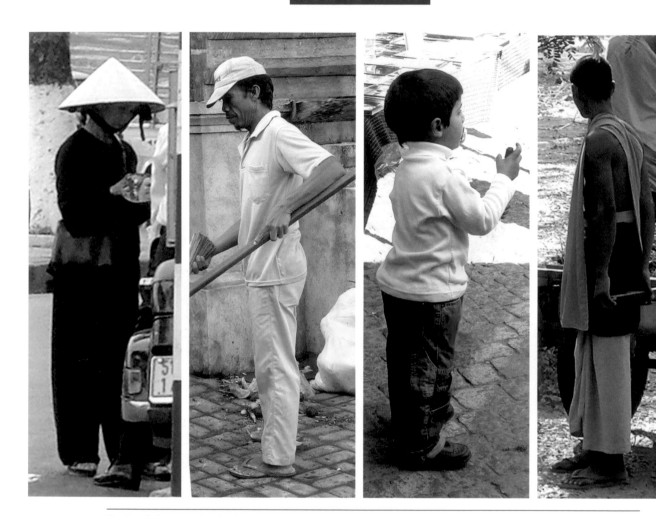

Each of these individuals, no matter the age, stands in a relaxed pose yet does not collapse or overarch the spine.

- Stand on active feet with knees rotating outward.
- Bow slightly at the hips until you can see your ankles (anchor the pelvis).
- Relax your belly.
- Release the chest down and in while lifting your back (power button).
- Roll one shoulder at a time onto the top of the rib cage (fasten your shoulders).

- Drop your chin slightly. Do a neck sweep, being sure to pause and release any tension as it arises.
- Breathe in a natural and relaxed way.

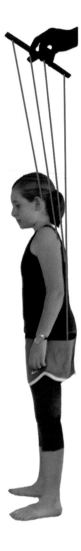

It helps to remember that the natural head is slightly forward. This may feel very odd at first, especially if you are accustomed to having your chin lifted and your head pulled back.

Standing Shortcut
- Stand on active feet.
- Look down at your feet.
- Do a neck sweep.
- Relax.

TAKE YOURSELF FOR A WALK

Nothing works better for relearning natural walking than using a strap or scarf to take yourself for a walk. Turning yourself, literally, into a puppet on a string tips the pelvis forward, turns the rib cage wheel forward, elongates the spine, and shifts your weight into the front of your body with your head leading. A long yoga strap with a buckle or clasp is ideal for this. You can use a scarf too if it is long enough to tie around your middle with enough leftover to be held overhead.

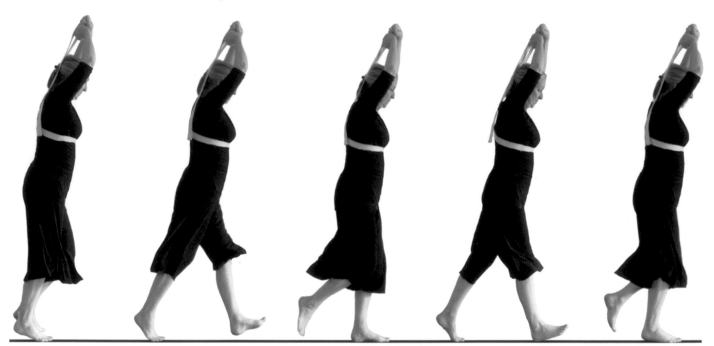

Gather a strap or long scarf and position it around your middle as shown here.

- Begin by placing the strap around the bottom of your rib cage (it can be easier to secure it in the front first and then turn it around so that the buckle or knot is in the center of your back). Take hold of the loose end and hold it above your head.
- Standing with your feet a few inches apart, draw the strap over your head and forward, using a strong enough pull to force you to start walking.

- Let the steps you take be relatively fast-paced, so that you don't have time to think about what you are doing. Just keep pulling yourself along, surrendering to the experience of almost falling forward.
- Your entire body becomes a wheel turning forward as the weight from above shifts onto the landing foot and the toes of the back foot push off against the floor, propelling the body forward. As soon as all the weight is on the front foot it shifts to being the pushing-off foot that drives the other foot and leg forward.

These words will make more sense after you've experienced this yourself. Take yourself for a walk now. You can also picture imaginary strings on your sitz bones, drawing the pelvis behind you, putting all the action for walking into your legs and buttocks, where it belongs. The best part of using an actual puppet string in this way is that after you've practiced with this a bit you can just *imagine* that a strap is tied around your middle for natural walking to happen on its own. Remember the feeling of the strap tipping your pelvis forward and lengthening your entire torso. You can experience this in your body in almost everything you do.

SITTING DOWN AND BENDING TO SIT

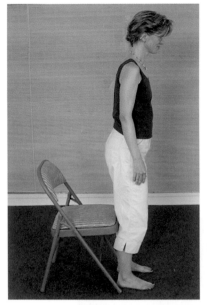
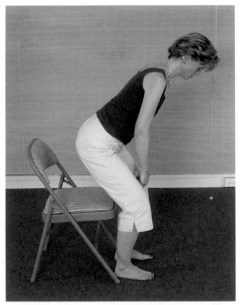
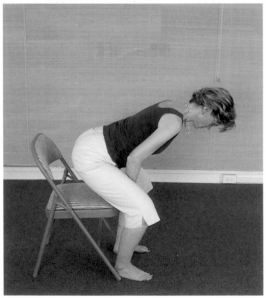
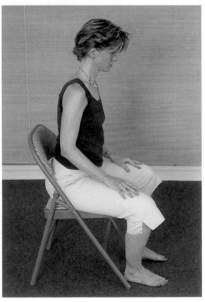

As with standing, walking, and bending, the back remains straight when sitting down.

- Stand with the back of your legs just touching the edge of a chair.
- Bend your knees outward as your sitz bones slide out behind you. Do not lift your sitz bones up behind you as this will tighten your back.

- The back of the neck remains long as you place the pubic bone and sitz bones on to the chair.
- Turn on the power button as you bring the upper body into an upright sitting position.
- Roll the shoulders, one at time, on top of the rib cage, then softly draw your chin up the front of your throat (neck sweep).
- Relax the belly and observe the breath.

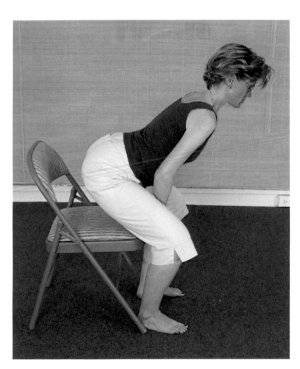

When bending, be sure you do not lift your chin or your chest as pictured here. This will cause your lower back to arch and the back of your neck to shorten and compress.

Sitting Down Shortcut

- Bend knees outward.
- Sitz bones extend behind.
- Spine remains long and straight.
- Use bending legs to lower onto chair.
- Bring torso to vertical.

SITTING TO MEDITATE

Setting up the pelvis to support an elongated spine is important when meditating, because unnecessary tension in the body can cause problems while meditating.

Meditators benefit greatly from knowing how to align the skeleton, often discovering that their meditation practice is greatly enhanced when they learn how

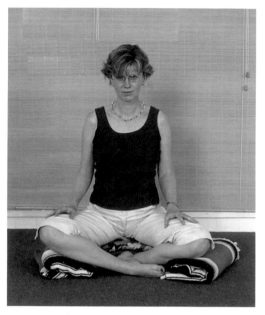

The most common position for meditation is to sit cross-legged on an anchored pelvis with the sitz bones elevated on a cushion or folded blanket. Imagine your pubic bone falling forward off the edge of the surface on which you are sitting. If your knees don't rest on the floor, place a rolled blanket or cushion under each knee to allow the hips to relax. Over time the hips will gradually release and open.

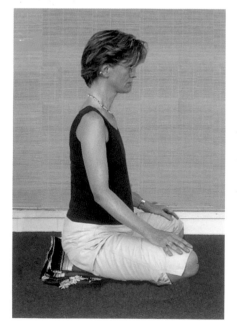

The cushion you sit on can be higher than the one pictured here if this helps your knees to come to rest on the floor.

to do this. A common misperception is that meditation is about transcending or overcoming the body. Let the body be the anchor and the crux of your inward focus.

- Anchor the pelvis on a cushion or chair, letting the front of the pelvis have weight.
- Relax your belly, experiencing your center of gravity in the abdomen.
- Release the chest down, as the middle of your back rises and opens behind you.
- Roll one shoulder at a time onto the top of the rib cage.
- Drop the chin and slide it slowly up the throat, lengthening the neck and relaxing all tension (neck sweep). Your chest stays down.
- Let the inner body (the skeleton) support you so that the outer body (everything else) relaxes.
- Observe the breath gently rising and falling away.

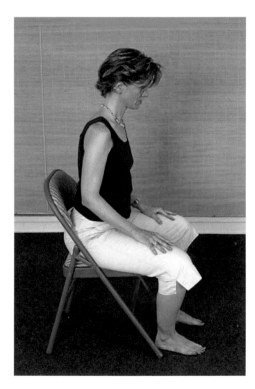

You can also sit in a chair with your feet flat on the floor. If you do sit in a chair, do not use the backrest but let a well-anchored pelvis provide support for the spine.

SLEEPING AND RESTING ON YOUR BACK

Lying flat on the floor or a bed rolls the rib cage backward and causes the lower back to arch. This interferes with being able to relax deeply. Supporting the head and shoulders with two soft pillows takes the arch out of the lumbar spine. In some cases you will need more than two pillows.

- Sit with knees bent so that when you roll down onto the pillows, the lower pillow comes to the bottom of the shoulder blades, and the upper pillow is just under the top edge of the shoulders. Resist any urge to tuck your butt.

- Press into the floor with both elbows, and lengthen your lower back toward the pillows. Your back will widen, and your chest will feel (momentarily) like it is collapsing.

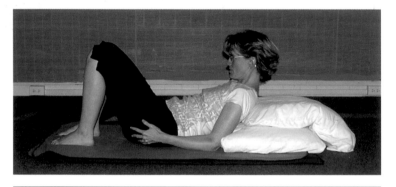

Be sure to use your elbows to hitch your back up behind you (power button) when lying down.

- Reach up with both hands on either side of the top pillow and roll the top pillow under so that your head is supported with the chin dropped slightly and the back of your neck is long (head wheel rolling forward). A small, very soft pillow works best for under the head.

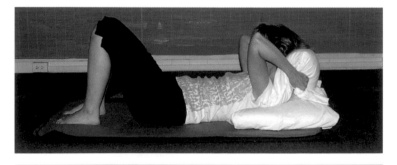

Notice how the pillow is folded to support the head.

- Let your shoulder blades slide down your back while keeping your chest from lifting as you do this.
- Surrender your weight into the pillows and the floor or bed underneath you. Become aware of the breath as it touches every part of your body, letting go of any tension with each exhalation.

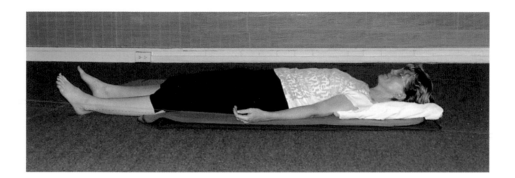

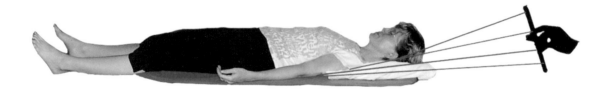

If you are comfortable and have lots of length through your entire spine, including your neck, with no arching in your lower back, you may be able to use only one pillow under your shoulders. This is discussed further in the relaxation segment of chapter 12, "Yoga on the Axis."

12

YOGA ON THE AXIS

YOGA HAS BECOME tremendously popular in recent years due in large part to the many benefits it offers. Yoga can build stamina and vitality, as well as an enhanced sense of well-being. It can cultivate a quality of awareness and a deepening ability to relax. For some, yoga (the meaning of which is "union") offers spiritual benefits, a sense of uniting with the divine, through a sense of merging with the oneness of all that is.

For some people, however, practicing yoga can lead to injury or pain. This is almost always the outcome of having misaligned bones while doing postures, or asanas, that are based on the modern, Western misunderstanding of "good" posture. This can happen while a distorted spine is being twisted, a misaligned hip is being opened, and a misfired muscle is being stretched. Sometimes the consequence of this is a day or two of feeling sore afterward, but done repetitively this can lead to more serious problems.

The good news is that yoga can be practiced in a way that conforms to the body's natural design. Not only that, doing yoga this way reinforces helpful new habits and accelerates an ability to inhabit the body more naturally in everything else we do.

The point of this approach is to allow flexibility to manifest itself by creating conditions that foster letting go. This can occur only when the underlying structural support is in place at the outset. A more authentic, lasting flexibility results from this, and more efficient movement patterns are introduced and reinforced in the body. This is different from imposing a temporary sort of flexibility on muscles that comes through repetitive stretching. In the same way that muscular strength gained from weight training disappears rapidly when the workouts cease, flexibility from stretching will last only as long as the stretching is repeated over and over again. Natural flexibility is balanced with a strong internal core that stabilizes an open, elongated spine and is the outcome of a recurring interplay between aligned bones and elastic muscles. This kind of flexibility is not only enduring, it is also our natural state. The instructions for the asana presented here are designed to reinforce these details.

Please review the "Try It On!" explorations on the pages listed on page 263 to be sure that you understand them. These form the basis for the steps that are applied in all the yoga asanas that follow. When standing, always begin by planting active feet, with your legs as vertical pillars and your knees and thighs rotating outward, away from each other. When sitting, take the time to establish the foundational support of your pelvis.

This approach to the practice of yoga is intended to reinforce the body's natural design that preserves the integrity of an elongated spine at all times. Doing any postures that work in opposition to this, such as rounding the spine in one direction or arching it in the other, are avoided. Thus we take great care here to maintain an essential partnership between the pelvis as the foundation and the rib cage as the nexus to a fully open and elongated spine. By maintaining this reciprocal relationship in all that we do, we remain connected to the body's innate home base and maintain a deeply solid core.

These postures are meant to be practiced with an awareness of remaining on "this side of the edge" in terms of encountering sensations of resistance or stretch. This could be described as delicately flirting with the sensations, encountering them as an experience to be explored with interest and respect. Rather than going for the stretch (or the "burn"), we invite a process of letting go. This occurs when softly exhaling while creating conditions of structural support. This skeletal support is the framework on which each asana is built and that aligns us, both literally and figuratively, with who we are as physical creatures and embodied presence. We don't open our tight hips by stretching them open but by reminding them, in positions of safety, how to be naturally free from stiffness and tension. The changes are gradual, yet they are significant and lasting.

Ultimately one doesn't need a physical practice of yoga for this to occur. We just need to inhabit the body in the natural way in all that we do. Either way, the changes will happen. The formal practice of yoga exercises, when done under the right conditions, however, can serve to enhance and accelerate this process and can come with a whole boatload of other benefits as well.

CHAIR POSE

Utkatasana

This pose reinforces the body's way of natural bending. When done according to these instructions it places the responsibility onto the feet and legs to provide support for an upper body that is relaxed and dynamic. Chair pose captures foundational elements of the practices of t'ai chi and qigong and other martial arts.

Prepare for the Posture

- Stand on active feet with your feet beneath your shoulders.
- Anchor the pelvis. Be sure the front of your thighs and your pubic bone are aiming behind you. Looking down you should be able to see the floor behind your heels.
- Exhale and turn on the power button. Maintain an engaged core as the breath rides gently over it.
- Do a feather soft neck sweep.

Move into the Posture

- Inhale into your back as you raise your arms, palms facing each other, out in front of you.
- Recharge the power button as you exhale, moving your hips behind you while bending your knees outward.
- Make sure your chest does not lift as you bend and that your back remains wide. This will stabilize your spine.
- To release from the pose exhale and press your feet deeply into the floor as the back of the rib cage rises to bring you to standing.
- Pay attention when coming up to be sure that your hips do not move forward of the axis, causing your pelvis to tuck.

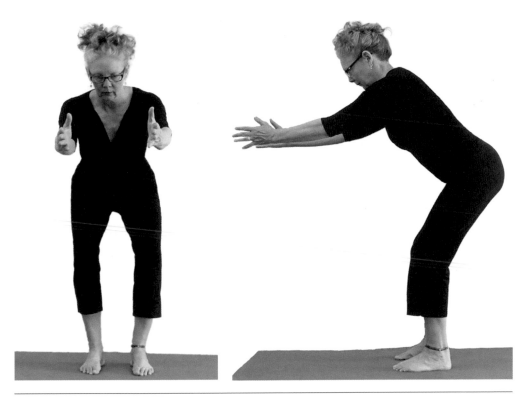

Notice how the back is straight and bending is from the hips and knees.

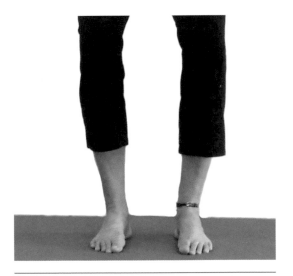

Your feet should be firmly planted as you rise.

TREE POSE

Vrksasana

Balance poses are more solidly rooted when our bones are aligned along the vertical axis.

Prepare for the Posture

- Stand on active feet, with heels tucked, in line with your shoulders.
- Anchor the pelvis. Move the thighs back so that the pubic bone is aiming behind your heels. Looking straight down you should be able to see the floor behind your heels.
- Exhale and turn on the power button, and maintain this engaged core as the breath rises and falls gently across it.

Moving into the Posture

- Place the right foot on the inside of the left thigh or your calf (not on the inside of the knee).
- Fasten the shoulders, then bring your arms up in front of you, palms facing each other. Lift your arms only as high as you are able to do without the chest rising or the back arching. The tops of the shoulders remain level and do not lift toward your ears.
- Your back is wide and rising, as if being held by a puppet string.
- Focus your gaze on one spot in front of you and let each inhalation fill your back.
- Exhale as you return your foot to the floor.
- Repeat from the beginning on the other side.

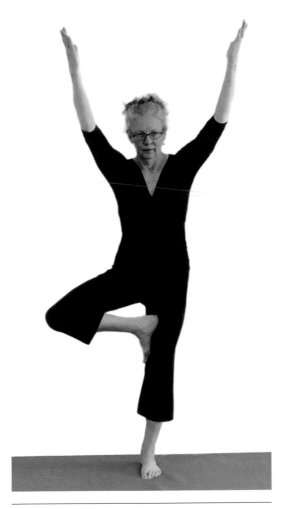

Notice how your stance is anchored, without unnatural lifting or stretching.

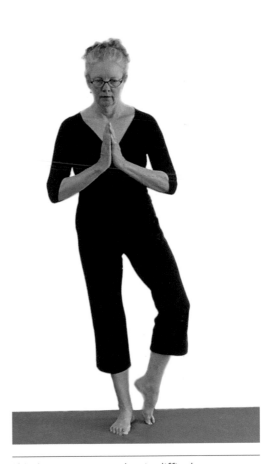

If balancing on one leg is difficult, you can build up to it gradually, first touching the toes of your lifted foot just barely on the floor.

TRIANGLE POSE (MODIFIED)

Trikonasana

Prepare for the Posture

- Stand with your feet wide apart (approximately as wide as your legs are long).
- Turn your left foot out 90 degrees, and your right foot in slightly toward the center. Line up the left heel with right heel.
- Anchor the pelvis. Place your hands on your thighs and guide them back until your pubic bone is aiming down and back behind your heels. Looking down you should be able to see behind your heels.
- Exhale and turn on the power button. Maintain the engaged core as the breath rides gently across it.

Move into the Posture

- Place your left hand in the crease of the left hip and gently guide your pelvis to the right as you exhale. The pelvis, torso, and head will all tip to the left as one continuous column.
- Bend the left knee *slightly*. Place the back of your arm on the front of your thigh. Do not lean into the arm or put weight on it.
- Rotate your left knee to the back. Your left foot will become more activated.
- Bring your right arm up overhead, palm facing forward, and fasten the shoulder blades onto the back of the rib cage.
- Do a feather soft neck sweep.
- Turn your head upward only as far as the neck remains soft and relaxed.
- Focus on the breath as it gently fills your back.
- Exhale to release the pose by pressing your feet deeply into the floor as the right hand rises farther upward to bring the body back up to standing.
- Repeat from the beginning on the other side.

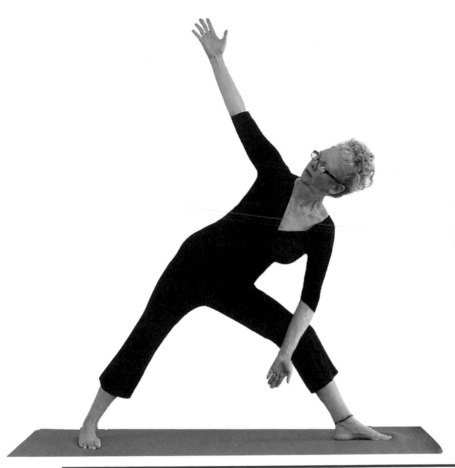

Be sure to keep the core engaged while performing the exercise.

WARRIOR II

Virabhadrasana

Warrior II pose, with bones aligned along the vertical axis, puts the responsibility into the feet and legs to provide unshakeable support for an upper body that can be free of tension and struggle. This is the pose of the peaceful warrior, receptive and open, while firmly planted and solidly strong.

Prepare for the Posture

- Stand with your feet wide apart (approximately as wide as your legs are long).
- Turn the toes of your left foot out to the left and your right foot in toward the center. Line up the left heel with the right heel.
- Anchor the pelvis. Be sure the front of your thighs and your pubic bone are aiming back, not forward (see images on facing page). Looking straight down you should be able to see the floor behind your heels. Do not actively lift your sitz bones, because this will tighten your lower back.
- Activate your feet by rotating your knees away from the center.

Move into the Posture

- Exhale and raise your arms out to the sides, shoulder level.
- Exhale and turn on the power button. Maintain the engaged core as the breath rides gently across it, filling and widening. This will relax your back and free your upper body from having to struggle.
- On the next exhalation bend the left knee and sink the pelvis toward the floor. Adjust as necessary to bring your left knee directly over your left ankle and aim it toward the outside of the foot.
- Do a feather soft neck sweep.
- Fasten the shoulder blades onto the back of the rib cage.
- Release from the pose by exhaling as you press your feet deeply into the floor, straightening the knee.
- Repeat from the beginning on the other side.

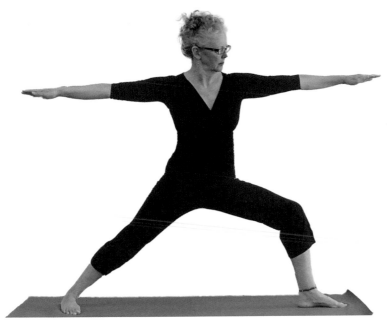

Your upper body should rest easily over your anchored pelvis and feet.

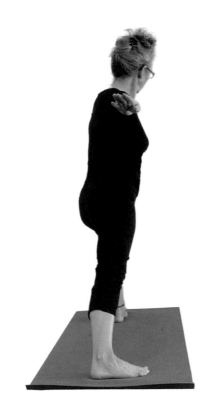

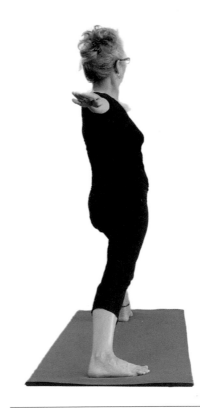

On the axis

Off the axis

GARDEN GATE POSE

Parighasana

Prepare for the Posture

- Kneel on a blanket. Be sure entire shin bone is on the blanket (see photo below). Use a second blanket to support your ankle, if necessary.
- Step the left leg to the side with knee bent and foot flat on the floor. The heel of the left foot is lined up with the right knee.
- Anchor the pelvis by aiming the pubic bone back.
- Place the left wrist on the inner left thigh, applying a small amount of pressure.
- Bring the right arm out in front, palm facing in.
- Turn on the power button.
- Fasten the shoulder blades.
- Do a neck sweep.
- Bring the right arm up, keeping the chest and shoulder blade in place.
- Inhale.

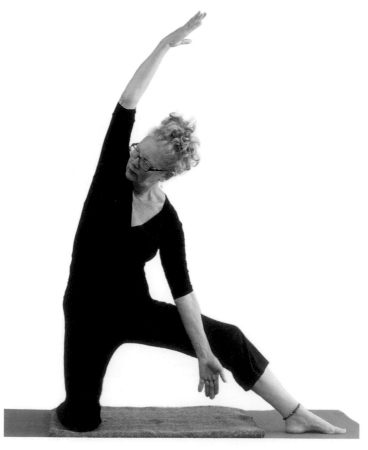

Be mindful of your alignment so as not to lean back during this pose.

Move into the Posture

- Slide the bottom of the rib cage to the right, maintaining the fullness in your back.
- Exhale and engage the power button (transversus abdominus) to prevent the bottom front ribs from rolling up as you turn your torso away from your left leg.
- Breathe into your lower back throughout the pose.
- Exhale to release from the pose, bringing your torso upright and your right arm down.
- Repeat from the beginning on the other side.

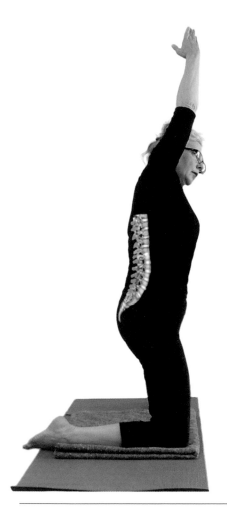

On the axis

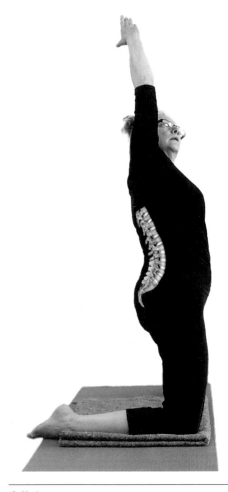

Off the axis

SPHINX POSE

Salamba Bhujangasana

Even a beginning back bend like this one can result in injury when the back arches and the spine is compressed. When the relationship between the pelvis and the rib cage is stabilized, Sphinx pose is beneficial in reinforcing the deep core of support for a long, open spine. Indeed, this is precisely what infants, when lying on their stomachs, are busily doing in the earliest months of their lives.

Prepare for the Posture

- Lie on your stomach with your elbows on the floor in line with your shoulders, palms down.
- Take a moment to feel the weight of your body resting on the floor.
- Your legs are extended straight behind you, side by side, with your feet close together.
- Press the tops of your feet into the floor as you roll the backs of the thighs away from each other so that the heels separate. This anchors the pelvis and opens the sacrum.
- Fasten the shoulder blades into place. With the arms in this position the elbows will draw in toward the body. This is similar to the wall push-ups, in the "Exercises to Save the Shoulders" on page 116, which secure the shoulder blades into place and strengthen stabilizing muscles in a balanced way.

Move into the Posture

- Turn on the power button as you begin to gently push the entire body into the floor. You will feel your core engage more deeply as the upper body rises away from the floor.

- Draw the hands and arms back as if pulling the floor toward you. Sense the back widening and the spine elongating as the base of the skull extends forward, moving the head with it.
- The breath remains gentle and soft as you hold the pose.
- To release, exhale as you lower your chest and head to the floor and relax your arms.

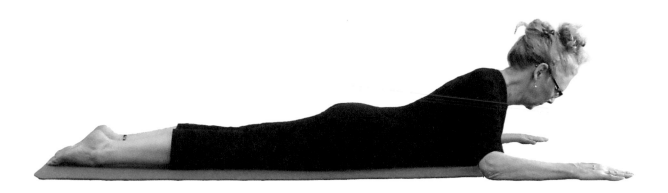

Notice that your back does not arch as your torso rises.

SEATED SPINAL TWIST

Supta Matsyendrasana

Spinal twists reinforce natural movement and stimulate the nervous system when done with an aligned spine. This twist can also be done sitting on a blanket, but we show it done sitting in a chair here as a way you can do this while taking a break from computer work.

Prepare for the Posture

- Sit on a chair with a level seat, your feet flat on the floor. Let your knees relax open.
- Anchor your pelvis on the chair.
- Turn on the power button.
- Fasten the shoulder blades.
- Do a feather soft neck sweep.

Move into the Posture

- Exhale and recharge the power button as the right sitz bone slides back and the left sitz bone slides forward. The pelvis, torso, and head rotate to the right as one continuous column.
- Place your right hand on the back of the seat and the back of your left hand to the outside of your right knee. Turning your palm forward will open the front of the shoulder and keep the shoulder blade in place. Do not use the pressure of your hands to push or pull yourself any farther.

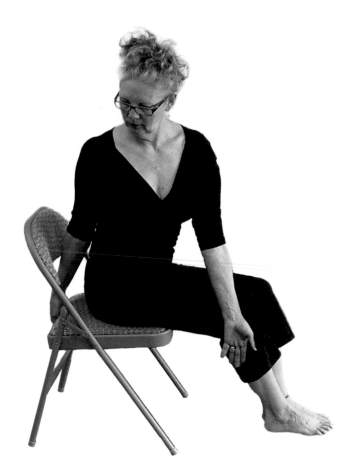

Let any deepening of the pose come from the letting go that occurs within the body and mind.

- Continue to use each exhalation to engage the front of the pelvis dropping, the back of the rib cage rising, and the center of the core releasing to the right.
- To release, exhale slowly to unwind and face forward.
- Repeat from the beginning on the other side.

RELAXATION—CORPSE POSE

Savasana

Prepare for the Posture

- Fold one or two blankets, as pictured, so that the first level supports the shoulder blades and a slightly higher level supports the neck and head.
- Lie down with your knees placed over a bolster or pillow.
- Clasp your hands behind the base of your head.
- Draw your elbows away from you as the neck lengthens.
- Be sure to turn on the power button and engage the core as you do this.

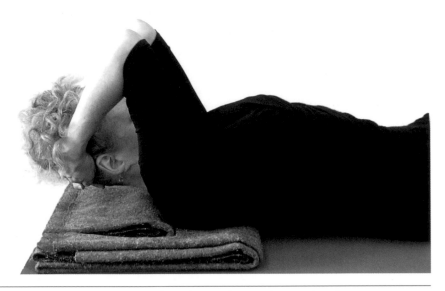

Lengthen with your neck rather than pulling with your hands.

- Your pubic bone extends away from the navel, as your lower back slides along the floor toward your head.

Move into the Posture

- Lay your head down onto the blanket, keeping the length in the neck as you do so, and relax your arms to your sides, palms facing up.
- Fasten your shoulder blades onto the back of the rib cage without letting your chest lift up.

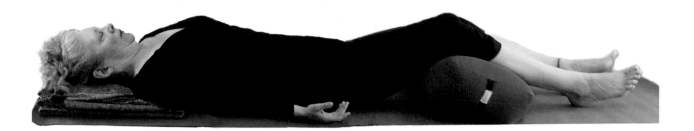

Feel the utter relaxation of lying with an aligned and supported core.

- Exhale and sense your head, trunk, arms, and legs all relaxing as you surrender the weight of your body into the earth.
- Follow the gentle rise and fall of the breath as you rest here for five to fifteen minutes, if possible.

Note: If you are comfortable and have lots of length through your entire spine, you may be able to use only one blanket under your shoulders. If your back is arched or you feel any discomfort, use two blankets. If this is still not completely comfortable, refer to chapter 11 for how to use extra pillows or blankets for supporting a relaxed spine.

As mentioned before, be sure to use your elbows to hitch your back up behind you (power button) when lying down. This is far more beneficial than trying to rest in a position that reinforces unnatural patterns.

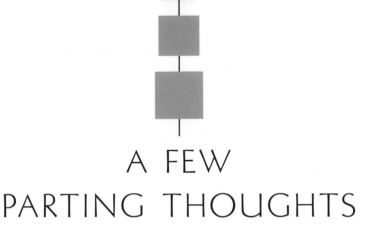

A FEW
PARTING THOUGHTS

- Don't try too hard. Trust that your body will know what to do as you put these guidelines into practice.

- Nevertheless, keep practicing as often as you can.

- Notice if you have a tendency when sitting to shift back and forth between being a tense dog and a sad dog: when your chest lifts up, your butt goes out, and while your chest drops down, your butt tucks under. Learn to be the happy dog in the middle, with your butt out and your chest down.

- Inhabit the body with the mind by thinking in terms of passive verbs (rise, drop, sink) instead of active verbs (push, pull, lift).

- Engage with the earth with your body dropping down and rising back up (Newton's third law).

- Let your pelvis have weight. Drop roots into the earth. Be grounded.

- Think length through your spine with space between the vertebrae, equal in the front and the back.

- Regularly pause and park the pelvis, then feel your back rising behind you.

- Initiate movements from your feet and pelvis aiming back and down as your back and torso elongate upward.

- Think softness, openness, and freedom in your joints.

- Feel boundaries melting. Feel inner and outer merging.

- Relax your jaw and neck and drop your chin.

- Let the soft breath rise and fall away from a place low in the belly. Experience the breath in your back more than your front. This will aid alignment and presence.

- When in doubt—about anything—relax your belly.

- Fall in love with your body and the peace to be found within.

- Smile often.

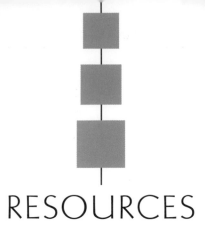

RESOURCES

The people listed here all teach principles of natural alignment based on the innate human design discovered by all naturally developing babies and toddlers and described in the pioneering work of Noelle Perez. Different teachers bring their own unique insights and talents to sharing this information. No distinction is made here between the effectiveness or value of these differing approaches, because one person may more readily integrate one approach while another way of learning this fits best with someone else. The intention in making this list available is to provide opportunities for learning natural alignment to as many people in as many locations as possible. Because of space considerations I have included only those teachers with websites.

TEACHERS OF NATURAL ALIGNMENT

Within the United States

Kathleen Porter
Portland, Oregon
Center for Natural Alignment
www.NaturalAlignment.com
kathleen@naturalalignment.com
503-505-1996

Jean Couch
Palo Alto, California
The Balance Center
www.BalanceCenter.com
jean@balancecenter.com
650-856-2000

Dana Davis
Petaluma, California
Sonoma Body Balance
www.SonomaBodyBalance.com
dana@sonomabodybalance.com
707-658-2599

Thea Sawyer
San Jose, California
www.LiveInBalance.com
thea@liveninbalance.com
408-489-9436

Mary Sinclair
Columbus, Ohio
www.MarySinclairBalance.com
mary@marysinclairbalance.com
614-906-0260

Kim Thompson
Gaithersburg, Maryland
www.OptimizedMovement.com
kim@optimizedmovement.com
301-519-9532

Jay Bunker, D.C.
Berkeley, California
www.DrJayBunker.com
jaybunker@earthlink.net
510-528-3058

Angelika Thusius
Kentro Body Balance
Ashland, Oregon
www.KentroBodyBalance.com
kentrobodybalance@gmail.com
541-944-1942

Lisa Ann McCall
Bend, Oregon
McCall Body Balance
www.mccallmethod.com
lisaann@mccallmethod.com
214-957-0234

Esther Gokhale
Palo Alto, California
The Gohkale Method
www.egwellness.com
info@egwellness.com
650-324-3244

Nora Braverman
New York, New York
www.NoraBraverman.com
nora@norabraverman.com
646-784-0748

Outside the United States

Noelle Perez (and associated teachers)
Paris, France
L'Institut Superieur d'Aplomb
www.isaplomb.org

YOGA TAUGHT IN
NATURAL ALIGNMENT

Moline Whitson
Portland, Oregon
www.HarmonyYogaPortland.com

Dana Davis
Petaluma, California
www.SonomaBodyBalance.com

Morgan Bursiel
Fairbanks, Alaska
www.InteriorYoga.com

Jean Farmwald
Half Moon Bay, California
www.BalanceCenter.com

Nora Braverman
New York, New York
www.NoraBraverman.com

Janet Cook
Palo Alto, California
www.BalanceCenter.com

Jenn Sherer
Palo Alto, California
www.BalanceCenter.com

Beth Greenfield Rodgers
Berkeley, California
www.4thStreetYoga.com

Laura Albrecht
Santa Cruz, California
www.YogaWithLaura.Weebly.com

COMPLEMENTARY APPROACHES
AND MODALITIES

Mindfulness Training

The cultivation of mindfulness is invaluable in partnership with retraining the body to be naturally aligned as well as generally living with greater awareness. A growing number of centers offer classes and retreats in mindfulness meditation in cities and towns everywhere. An Internet search will help you find one in your area.

Alexander Technique

Developed by F. M. Alexander more than a century ago, the Alexander technique has helped thousands of people learn how to inhabit their bodies in a more natural, relaxed way. This technique shares a number of important details in common with natural alignment and places emphasis on awareness and conscious remapping of unhelpful habits. Alexander technique has been particularly popular among musicians and actors. If you are unable to find a teacher of natural alignment in your area you may have more success locating an Alexander technique teacher to work with you.

American Society for the Alexander Technique
www.amsatonline.org/teachers

Movement, Exercise, and Martial Arts

A number of disciplines, some quite ancient, provide the benefit of reinforcing natural alignment (when done correctly). These also promote easeful, natural movement and deep relaxation. These include qigong, t'ai chi, aikido, kung fu, and kendo. It is important that teachers of t'ai chi and qigong have been properly trained to understand that the instruction for tucking does not mean tucking the tailbone by rotating the pelvis backward or aiming the pubic bone toward the navel. Martial arts masters from traditional training understand that *tuck* means shifting an anteverted pelvis forward in space, by shifting the weight of the whole body forward through the feet.

An Internet search will easily direct you to teachers of these modalities in your area.

USEFUL TOOLS

The Wedge

This is a small, portable, wedge-shaped cushion that helps park the pelvis in the anchored, anteverted position for comfortable sitting anywhere. It can be used at a desk, in a car, on a plane, in a classroom, or at a movie, concert, or lecture. It is available from Natural Posture Solutions, LLC (www.NaturalPostureSolutions.com).

Comfy Shoulder Band

Comfy secures the shoulders in place and can be used while working at a computer or while sitting in meditation. It also functions as a training tool, reminding the body how to bend naturally and where home base is for the shoulders even when the band is no longer in use. It is also available from Natural Posture Solutions, LLC (www.NaturalPostureSolutions.com).

NOTES

CHAPTER 1. DESIGN FOR LIFE

1. E. Volinn, "The Epidemiology of Low Back Pain in the Rest of the World: A Review of Surveys in Low- and Middle-Income Countries," *Spine* 22, no. 15 (August 1997): 1747–54.
2. Claudia Kalb, "The Great Back Debate," *Newsweek,* April 26, 2004.
3. Jay S. Olshansky, Bruce A. Carnes, and Robert N. Butler, "If Humans Were Built to Last," *Scientific American,* March 2001, 51–55.

CHAPTER 2.
ARCHITECTURE IN FLESH AND BONE

1. Barbara F. Lujan and Ronald J. White, "Focus 6," in *Human Physiology in Space* (Houston, Tex.: National Space Biomedical Research Institute), www.nsbri.org/HumanPhysSpace/index.html.
2. Buckminster Fuller, "Tensegrity," in *Portfolio and Art News Annual; No. 4,* ed. Alfred Frankfurter (New York: The Art Foundation Press, 1961), 112–26.
3. Mabel E. Todd, *The Thinking Body* (Hightstown, N.J.: Princeton Book Company, 1937), 59–60.

CHAPTER 3. THE CORE OF WELL-BEING

1. A. P. French, *Newtonian Mechanics,* The M.I.T. Introductory Physics Series (New York: W. W. Norton and Company, 1971), 123–24.

CHAPTER 4. MEET YOUR FEET

1. J. Robert McClintic, *Basic Anatomy and Physiology of the Human Body* (New York: John Wiley and Sons, Inc., 1980), 157–60.

CHAPTER 5.
WHEELS, BELLS, AND PUPPET STRINGS

1. David Wise and Rodney Anderson, *A Headache in the Pelvis, A New Understanding and Treatment for Chronic Pelvic Pain Syndromes,* 6th rev. ed. (Occidental, Calif.: National Center for Pelvic Pain Research, 2012), 80–82.

2. Tim Parks, *Teach Us to Sit Still: A Skeptics Search for Health and Healing* (Emmaus, Pa.: Rodale Press, 2011).

3. Tim Parks, e-mail message to author, June 28, 2011.

4. Mabel E. Todd, *The Thinking Body* (Hightstown, N.J.: Princeton Book Company, 1937), 40.

5. Ingo Ebersberger, Dirk Metzler, Carsten Schwarz, and Svante Pääbo, "Genomewide Comparison of DNA Sequences between Humans and Chimpanzees," *American Journal of Human Genetics* 70, no. 15 (June 2002): 1490–97.

CHAPTER 6.
AN EXPLODING CRISIS IN CHILDREN'S HEALTH

1. "Attention Deficit/Hyperactivity Disorder Statistics," Centers for Disease Control and Prevention, CDC website, December 12, 2011, www.cdc.gov/ncbddd/adhd/data.html.

2. Roger W. Sperry, "The Future of Psychology: Remarks on Presentation of Lifetime Contribution Award, 1993," *American Psychologist* 50, no. 7 (1995): 505–6.

3. Jean Liedloff, *The Continuum Concept* (Cambridge, Mass.: Da Capo Press, 1986), 47–51.

4. "Health Information & Media—SIDS: Back to Sleep Campaign," National Institute of Child Health and Human Development, last updated September 15, 2009, www.nichd.nih.gov/sids/winter.cfm?from=women.

5. L. C. Argenta, L. R. David, J. A. Wilson, and W. O. Bell, "An Increase in Infant Cranial Deformity with Supine Sleeping Position," *Journal of Craniofacial Surgery* 7 (1996): 5–11.

6. Joanne E. Flanagan, Rebecca Landa, Anjana Bhat, and Margaret Bauman, "Head Lag Infants at Risk for Autism: A Preliminary Study," *The American Journal of Occupational Therapy* 66 (2012): 577–85.

7. Jonathan W. Jantz, Christopher D. Blosser, Lynne A Fruechting, "A Motor Milestone Change Noted with a Change in Sleep Position," *Pediatrics & Adolescent Medicine* 151, no. 6 (June 1997): 565–68.

8. "Autism and Developmental Disabilities Monitoring (ADDM) Network," Centers for

Disease Control and Prevention, CDC website, www.cdc.gov/ncbddd/autism/addm
.html (accessed March 12, 2012).

9. Joyce R. MacKinnon, Samuel Noh, Judith Lariviere, Ann MacPhail, Diane Allan, and Deborah Laliberte, "A Study of Therapeutic Effects of Horseback Riding for Children with Cerebral Palsy," *Physical and Occupational Therapy in Pediatrics* 15, no. 1 (1995): 17–34; Bonnie Lutz, "Clinical Implications of Hippotherapy," Chapman University, August 2, 2010, www.specialspirit.org/uploads/3/9/3/6/3936974/why_horses.pdf; and Ann MacPhail, Janice Edwards, Jane Golding, et al., "Trunk Postural Reactions in Children with and without Cerebral Palsy during Therapeutic Horseback Riding," *Pediatric Physical Therapy* 10, no. 4 (Winter 1998): 143–47.

10. M. M. Bass, C. A. Duchowny, and M. M. Llabre, "The Effect of Therapeutic Horseback Riding on Social Functioning in Children with Autism," *Journal of Autism and Developmental Disorder* 39, no. 9 (September 2009): 1261–67.

11. William Benda, Nancy H. McGibbon, and Kathryn L. Grant, "Improvements in Muscle Symmetry in Children with Cerebral Palsy After Equine-Assisted Therapy," *Journal of Alternative and Complementary Medicine* 9, no. 6 (December 2003): 817–25.

12. Susan Greenland, *The Mindful Child: How to Help Your Kid Manage Stress and Become Happier, Kinder, and More Compassionate* (New York: Simon and Schuster, 2010), 15–19.

CHAPTER 8. PREGNANT WITH POSSIBILITIES

1. Jill Schiff Boissonnault and Mary Jo Blaschak, "Incidence of Diastasis Recti Abdominis During the Childbearing Year," *Physical Therapy* 68, no. 7 (1988): 1082–86.

CHAPTER 9. IN FITNESS OR IN HEALTH?

1. J. P. Koplan, D. S. Siscovick, and G. M. Goldbaum, "The Risks of Exercise: A Public Health View of Injuries and Hazards," *Public Health Reports* 100, no. 2 (1985): 189–95.

2. D. M. W. De Coverley Veale, "Exercise Dependence," *British Journal of Addiction* 82, no. 7 (July 1987): 735–40.

3. D. W. Evans and L. C. Lum, "Hyperventilation: An Important Cause of Pseudoangina," *Lancet* 309, no. 8004 (January 1977): 155–57.

4. Susan E. Brown, "Rethinking Osteoporosis," *The Center for Better Bones Blog,* March 14, 2012, www.betterbones.com/osteoporosis/osteoporosis-statistics.aspx#spinalfracture.

5. Douglas C. Bauer, "Bisphosphonate Use and Atypical Femoral Fractures," *Journal of Clinical Endocrinology and Metabolism* 95, no. 12 (December 2010): 5207–9.

6. M. I. Weintraub, "Beauty Parlor Stroke Syndrome: Report of Five Cases," *Journal of the American Medical Association* 269, no. 16 (1993): 2085–86.

7. Tara Parker-Pope, "Stroke Rising among Young People," New York Times Blog, February 10, 2011, http://well.blogs.nytimes.com/2011/02/10/stroke-rising-among-young-people.

CHAPTER 10. BEYOND THE PHYSICAL

1. Carolyn Butler, "Meditation and Mindfulness May Give Your Brain a Boost," The Washington Post Blog, February 14, 2011, www.washingtonpost.com/wp-dyn/content/article/2011/02/14/AR2011021405973.html.

2. Carolyn Schatz, "Mindfulness Meditation Improves Connections in the Brain," Harvard Medical School Health Blog, April 8, 2011, www.health.harvard.edu/blog/mindfulness-meditation-improves-connections-in-the-brain-201104082253.

3. Anodea Judith, *Eastern Body, Western Mind: Psychology and the Chakra System as a Path to the Self* (Berkeley, Calif.: Celestial Arts, 1996), 5.

INDEX

BOOKS OF RELATED INTEREST

The New Rules of Posture
How to Sit, Stand, and Move in the Modern World
by Mary Bond

Balancing Your Body
A Self-Help Approach to Rolfing Movement
by Mary Bond

Rolfing
Reestablishing the Natural Alignment and Structural Integration
of the Human Body for Vitality and Well-Being
by Ida P. Rolf, Ph.D.

Trigger Point Self-Care Manual
For Pain-Free Movement
by Donna Finando, L.Ac., L.M.T.

Acupressure Taping
The Practice of Acutaping for Chronic Pain and Injuries
by Hans-Ulrich Hecker, M.D., and Kay Liebchen, M.D.

The Therapeutic Yoga Kit
Sixteen Postures for Self-Healing through Quiet Yin Awareness
by Cheri Clampett and Biff Mithoefer

No-Risk Abs
A Safe Workout Program for Core Strength
by Blandine Calais-Germain

Five Point Touch Therapy
Acupressure for the Emotional Body
by Pierre-Noël Delatte, M.D.

INNER TRADITIONS • BEAR & COMPANY
P.O. Box 388
Rochester, VT 05767
1-800-246-8648
www.InnerTraditions.com

Or contact your local bookseller